WALL PILATES

TO LOSE WEIGHT

KRISTEN PAYTON

TABLE OF CONTENTS

WHAT DOES THIS BOOK INCLUDE? 7

BASIC FUNDAMENTAL PRINCIPLES 9

DIFFERENCES BETWEEN WALL PILATES AND TRADITIONAL PILATES 10

PHYSICAL, MENTAL, AND EMOTIONAL BENEFITS 11

HOW TO INCREASE THE LEVEL OF DIFFICULTY OF THE EXERCISES 15

1 - TORSION WITH SUPPORT 16

2 - WALL SITTING POSITION 18

3 - HIP FLEXOR STRETCHING 20

4 - WALL SQUAT + KICK BACK 22

5 - SINGLE LEG GLUTE BRIDGE 24

6 - OPENING WITH LATERAL MOMENTUM STANDING 26

7 - SCISSORS 28

8 - DYNAMIC TORSION OF THE LEGS 30

9 - CHAIR ON THE WALL + ARM CIRCLE 32

10 - MOUNTAIN CLIMBER TO THE WALL 34

11 - FROM PLANK TO UPWARD STRETCHING 36

12 - TRICEPS PUSH UP TO THE WALL + KNEE RAISE 38

13 - HIP THRUST TO THE WALL WITH STATIC STOP 40

14 - CALF RAISES TO THE WALL 42

15 - RUSSIAN TWIST 44

16 - REVERSE CRUNCH TO THE WALL 46

17 - UNILATERAL GLUTE BRIDGE TO THE WALL 48

18 - KNEE TO CHEST + KICK BACK 50

19 - UNILATERAL DYNAMIC STRETCHING 52

20 - BULGARIAN SQUAT 54

21 - SEATED FORWARD STRETCH-OUTSTRETCHED ARMS 56

22 - TOUCH OPPOSITE TOES - BACK TO THE WALL 58

23 - FROG STRETCH 60

24 - WALK WHILE LYING DOWN AND THEN BRIDGE 62

25 - EXTENSION WITH SUPPORT ON THE WALL 64

26 - STANDING KNEE RAISE 66

27 - BUTTERFLY 68

28 - KNEE TO CHEST 70

29 - BUTTERFLY OPENING 72

30 - BRIDGE WITH KNEE TO CHEST 74

31 - STRETCHING LEGS SPLIT TO THE WALL 76

32 - BACK STRETCH TO THE WALL 78

33 - DYNAMIC EXTENSION TO THE WALL 80

34 - SCAPULAR RETRACTION & PROTRACTION 82

35 - ALTERNATE SHOULDER ROTATIONS 84

36 - ALTERNATE LEG FLEXION 86

37 - BACK STRETCHING AND ALTERNATE ARMS STRETCHING 88

38 - ARM RAISES WITH BOTTLE .... 9(

39 - PUSH BACK TO THE WALL 92

40 - CROSSED ARMS STRETCH 9

IMPORTANT INFORMATION BEFORE YOU START! .... 9(

28-DAY FAT BURNING CHALLENGE 97

TRACKING CHART 11

WHAT DOES THIS BOOK INCLUDE?

- THEORETICAL INTRODUCTION **PLUS** PRACTICAL ADVICE
- 40 EXERCISES WITH WRITTEN EXPLANATION AND STEP BY STEP PHOTOS

As promised, however, this is not all... we have included the following BONUSES:

1st BONUS: 40 VIDEO RECORDINGS OF THE EXERCISES INSIDE THE BOOK

2nd BONUS: 28-DAY FAT BURNING CHALLENGE

3rd BONUS: EBOOK ON INTERMITTENT FASTING

With the purchase of this book, you will have free access to:

1. THE MAIN THEORY ON WALL PILATES

2. PRACTICAL TIPS FOR BEGINNERS

3. 40 EXERCISES WITH:
- WRITTEN EXPLANATION
- STEP BY STEP ILLUSTRATIONS
- VIDEO RECORDINGS FOR EVERY SINGLE EXERCISE

4. 28-DAY FAT BURNING CHALLENGE

5. EBOOK INTERMITTENT FASTING

A significant amount of time and effort was dedicated to crafting this book. In a unique approach, we have included a video for each exercise to offer our customers a comprehensive guide. These videos allow you to easily observe and grasp the proper execution without having to spend excessive time reading the written instructions. Unlike many other Pilates books that may only contain 2-3 photos per exercise, making it challenging to interpret the correct movements and increasing the risk of injuries.

Moreover, with this book, you will enjoy complimentary access to all video recordings indefinitely.

HOW TO DOWNLOAD YOUR BONUSES:

SCAN THE QR CODE:

Thank you for selecting our book and for endorsing the hard work and dedication that went into creating these supplementary resources. We are confident that you will discover immense value in this guide!

Minimize the risk of injury and download the step-by-step videos now!

BASIC FUNDAMENTAL PRINCIPLES

What is Wall Pilates?

Wall Pilates is an innovative discipline inspired by traditional Pilates, but with a unique twist of incorporating the wall as the primary tool. This new approach makes it accessible to everyone, allowing individuals to comfortably practice the exercises from home at any time.

Origins

Pilates was founded by Joseph Pilates at the dawn of the 20th century, revolutionizing the landscape of modern fitness. The primary objective of this practice is to enhance physical fitness while simultaneously lowering daily stress levels. By incorporating the wall, individuals can engage in exercises suitable for both novices and experts, as the movements can be customized according to individual starting points. Wall Pilates is perfect for busy individuals seeking to stay in shape and enhance their physique conveniently at home.

Main features

Each Wall Pilates exercise demands attention and precision; it is essential to stay focused on both movement and breathing. Within this book, you will discover a variety of exercises designed to tone and strengthen your muscles, with a special focus on the abdomen to help you maintain a straight back and balance throughout your entire range of motion. The key priority is to concentrate on executing each exercise correctly to prevent injuries. Additionally, upon purchasing this book, you will receive access to videos demonstrating each exercise to ensure proper form and address any concerns. Wall Pilates caters to individuals of all levels, as it offers the flexibility to modify each movement and customize the routine according to your personal physical condition. These exercises are adaptable for increasing or decreasing intensity and difficulty. This innovative discipline retains all the advantages of traditional Pilates, including enhancing posture, correcting imbalances, and improving flexibility.

DIFFERENCES BETWEEN WALL PILATES AND TRADITIONAL PILATES

The primary difference between these two similar disciplines is the equipment they utilize. Traditional Pilates often requires specific tools, while the wall version only needs a simple mat to prevent slipping. The wall itself serves as the main tool, eliminating the need to purchase expensive and bulky equipment, allowing you to conveniently perform all exercises from your living room. Designed to utilize the wall as a support point, the exercises involve various inclinations and angles to adjust the level of difficulty.

The wide range of exercises achievable with just a wall and a mat enables comprehensive muscle training. For instance, "the bridge" exercise targets the glutes and core activation, while squats strengthen the quadriceps. Utilizing the wall facilitates prompt correction of exercise execution through downloadable videos.

Wall Pilates is suitable for individuals of all levels - the wall provides excellent balance support for beginners and increases exercise difficulty for more advanced practitioners. This adaptable discipline is gaining global popularity for its inclusivity, requiring no specific physical preparation and catering to individual needs, including those recovering from injuries.

PHYSICAL, MENTAL, AND EMOTIONAL BENEFITS

Physical benefits

Wall Pilates is ideal for strengthening the entire abdominal wall, as each exercise actively engages the core for balance and stability throughout the range of motion. This discipline includes exercises to improve flexibility, such as stretches, and tone muscles like glutes through squats, among others. The key physical benefits encompassed in this discipline are:

1. Posture Improvement:

The wall support aids in correcting postural alignment during exercises, promoting better body awareness that translates to improved posture beyond Pilates sessions.

2. Muscle Strength and Tonicity:

Wall resistance intensifies exercises, boosting muscle work intensity for enhanced tone and definition, especially in core, arm, and leg muscles.

3. Flexibility:

Wall Pilates significantly enhances flexibility by utilizing the wall as a supportive point for performing ideal pre- and post-workout muscle stretches, reducing injury risks.

4. Balance and Coordination:

The exercises and routines in this discipline enhance balance and coordination, with many movements requiring unilateral limb engagement and incorporating dynamic movements beyond static poses.

Mental and emotional benefits

In addition to physical improvements, wall Pilates offers positive psychological effects. Daily stress accumulation can significantly impact mental health, but regular practice of wall Pilates from this guide can promote emotional well-being, reducing stress and anxieties.

The main mental and emotional benefits include:

1. Stress reduction:

To perform the exercises correctly you need to stay concentrated and focused on the movement. This conscious, meditative focus occupies the mind and lets you temporarily put aside daily worries & relieve stress.

2. Greater self-confidence:

Many beginners feel a little uncomfortable when they go to a gym because they don't have much self-confidence and feel awkward when doing exercises for the first time.

Wall Pilates is different because you train at home, in complete privacy. By following the routines in this book you'll become good at them, building self-confidence.

The wall will also help support you while performing the exercises and will allow you to become familiar with the movement, limiting the risk of injuries. The most important thing is to focus on the mind-muscle connection. As time passes you will begin to see the first improvements and your self-esteem will grow more and more, alongside greater confidence in your physical abilities.

3. Cognitive Benefits:

This discipline is an ideal choice for those looking for a sport activity that has positive effects on both the body and the mind. It is a form of exercise that increases both physical and mental performance while also improving your cognitive and memory skills.

To carry out each exercise correctly you will first have to understand exactly how to perform it (don't forget to download the videos!!!), memorize the correct movement, and then repeat it. Obviously, you can consult the book at any time, but I urge you to make this effort from the beginning so as to fully exploit the potential of this discipline which, if carried out regularly, will improve your general well-being.

ADVICE BEFORE YOU START

How to integrate wall Pilates into your routine

Integrating Wall Pilates into your daily schedule may appear challenging but simply requires effective organization. The short training routines provided at the end of this guide demand minimal time commitment, necessitating analysis of your daily schedule to identify suitable time slots for this fulfilling practice amidst work and personal responsibilities. With proper organization and commitment, success in Wall Pilates is achievable, offering a rejuvenating experience with each session.

Tips for beginners

Are you a beginner and have never done a Pilates exercise in your life? Don't worry! Below you will find a short guide that will allow you to start with the first exercises today.

1. Understand the basic principles:

Before starting, it is essential to understand the fundamental principles of wall Pilates: concentration, control, focus, fluidity, precision and breathing. These principles are the basis of every movement and are necessary to derive the maximum benefit from this discipline. Don't underestimate them because they represent a fundamental starting point, especially if you're starting from scratch.

2. Get accustomed to the basic movements:

At the end of the book you will find training routines organized into the 28-day challenge. Before starting that I suggest taking a week to start familiarizing yourself with the exercises, understanding which movements you can and cannot perform correctly. It is not necessary to do an actual workout, but you can easily browse the book, watch the videos, and try to repeat the exercises in a slow and controlled way. This way you will prepare in advance for the 28-

day training program and will not have to waste time understanding the movement.

Start with the exercises that you think are simplest, make sure you can perform them correctly, then gradually begin to perform the more complex ones. I recommend starting with short sessions, gradually increase the duration and complexity of the exercises as you increase your strength and confidence. You will soon realize that once you understand the movement you will begin to have greater confidence and self-esteem, building motivation to keep going.

HOW TO INCREASE THE LEVEL OF DIFFICULTY OF THE EXERCISES

When you begin to have some experience with wall Pilates and you fully understand the movement of the exercises, you will be able to increase the level of difficulty with the use of different training strategies that will increase the intensity of the exercises. Your workouts will therefore become more complex and challenging! Follow these instructions to test yourself!

1. Create advanced exercises:

One of the quickest and easiest ways to make wall Pilates more complex is to experiment with new angles and levels of wall resistance. Many seemingly simple exercises can actually prove to be a real challenge! In fact, it is sufficient to change the angle of the movement to realize the change.

2. Combine basic exercises to create a circuit

To increase the intensity of your workouts I recommend you try this effective technique. Choose 2-3 basic exercises that you know you can perform correctly and try to do them in a row without a break. This method is ideal especially when you realize that you have fully understood the movement of certain exercises and would like to start increasing the difficulty. Then start creating sequences of exercises that target different areas of the body, experiment and identify the ones you consider most effective.

1 - TORSION WITH SUPPORT

BENEFITS

- Activation of the entire abdomen
- Stretching of the lower back

BREATHING

Inhale before starting the twist and exhale during the movement

HOW TO PERFORM THE EXERCISE

1 Sit on the mat with your feet flat against the wall

2 Keep your back straight

3 Raise your arms forming a 90-degree angle

4 Rotate your torso to the right and then to the left keeping your arms straight

TRICKS AND TIPS

Don't move too quickly. Control your execution by contracting your abs.

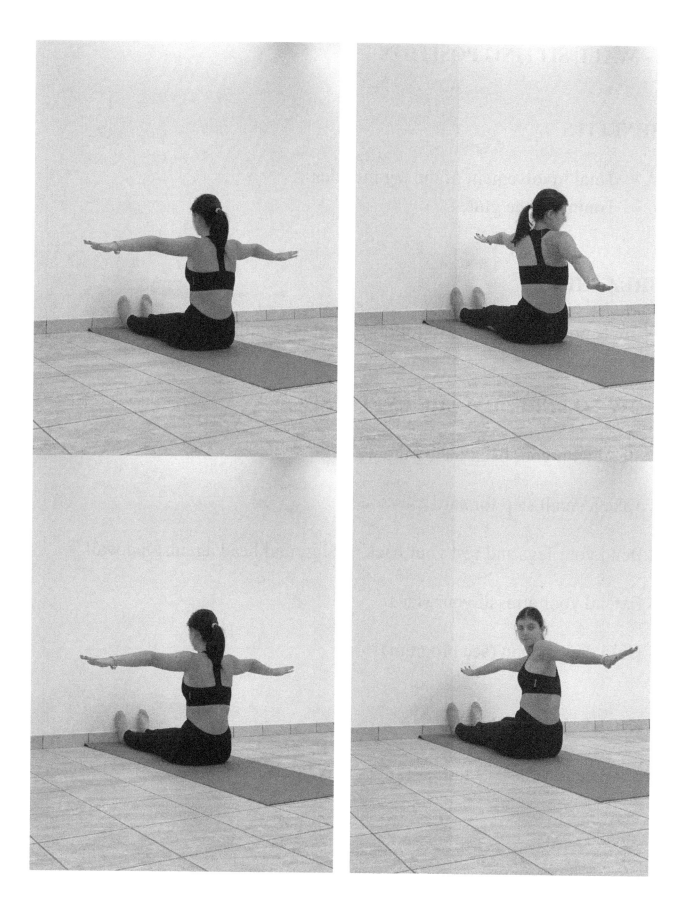

2 - WALL SITTING POSITION

BENEFITS

- Total involvement of the leg muscles
- Toning of the glutes

BREATHING

There is no particular rule to follow, maintain regular breathing.

HOW TO PERFORM THE EXERCISE

1 Stand with your back facing the wall

2 Take a small step forward

3 Bend your legs and rest your back, glutes, and head against the wall

4 Extend your arms at your sides

5 Hold the position (see program)

TRICKS AND TIPS

Do not bend your legs too far (knees max 90 degrees).

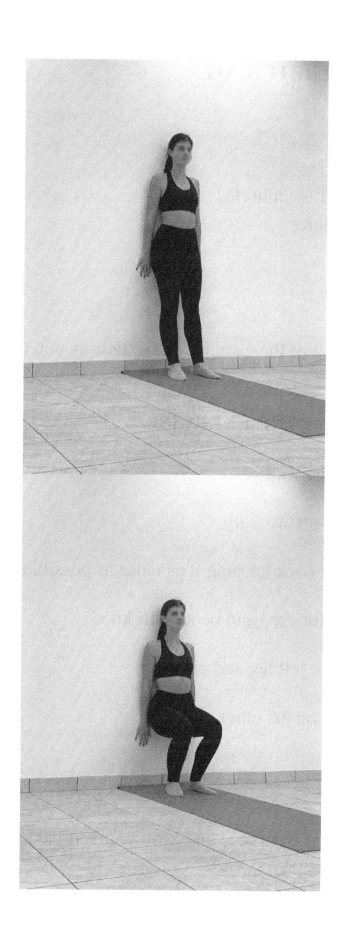

3 - HIP FLEXOR STRETCHING

BENEFITS

- Strengthening of leg muscles
- Toning of the glutes

BREATHING

Inhale at the beginning of the exercise and exhale as you bend your knee.

HOW TO PERFORM THE EXERCISE

1 Stand sideways to the wall

2 Put your right hand on the wall

3 Bring your right leg back keeping it as tense as possible

4 Bring your left leg forward and bend your knee

5 Use strength on your left leg and go up

6 Repeat the exercise on the other side

TRICKS AND TIPS

Place your left hand on your knee and keep yourself balanced with the help of your right hand resting on the wall.

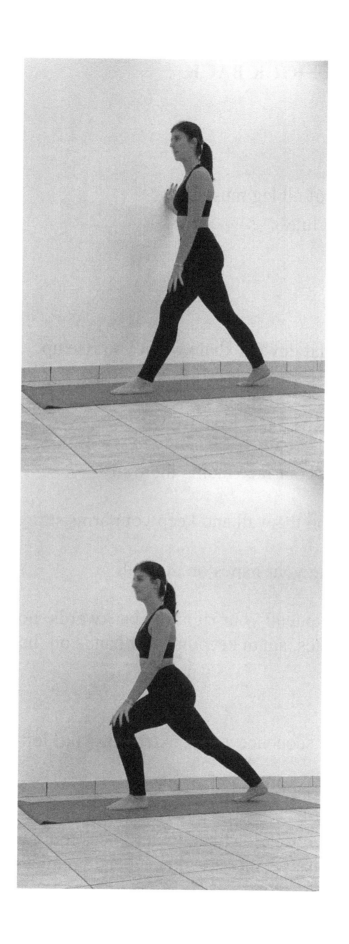

4 - WALL SQUAT + KICK BACK

BENEFITS

- Strengthening of all leg muscles
- Toning of the glutes

BREATHING

Inhale when you squat down, exhale when you rise up.

HOW TO PERFORM THE EXERCISE

1 Stand upright with your face facing the wall

2 Place your hands on the wall and keep your arms straight

3 Do a squat, keeping your hands on the wall

4 Rise back up and extend your right leg backwards, holding the position by contracting your glutes, again keeping your hands on the wall

5 Repeat the squat

6 Perform the above sequence again, extending your left leg

TRICKS AND TIPS

As you learn the exercise, don't bend your knees too much and keep pressure on your hands to assist. Increase knee bend gradually as you feel more comfortable with the exercise.

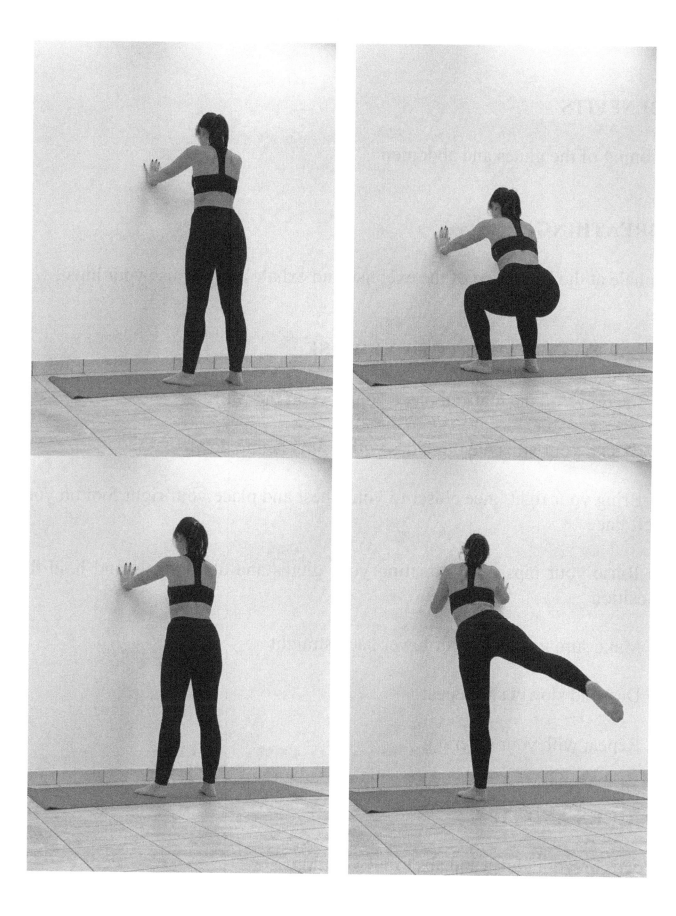

5 - SINGLE LEG GLUTE BRIDGE

BENEFITS

Toning of the glutes and abdomen

BREATHING

Inhale at the beginning of the exercise and exhale as you raise your hips.

HOW TO PERFORM THE EXERCISE

1 Lie down on the mat and place your feet on the wall

2 Extend your arms at your sides with palms facing down

3 Bring your right knee closer to your chest and place your right foot on your left knee

4 Raise your hips by contracting your glutes and abdominals and hold the position

5 Make sure you keep your lower back straight

6 Descend slowly and repeat

7 Repeat with your other leg

TRICKS AND TIPS

Focus on your glutes and abs to lift your hips.

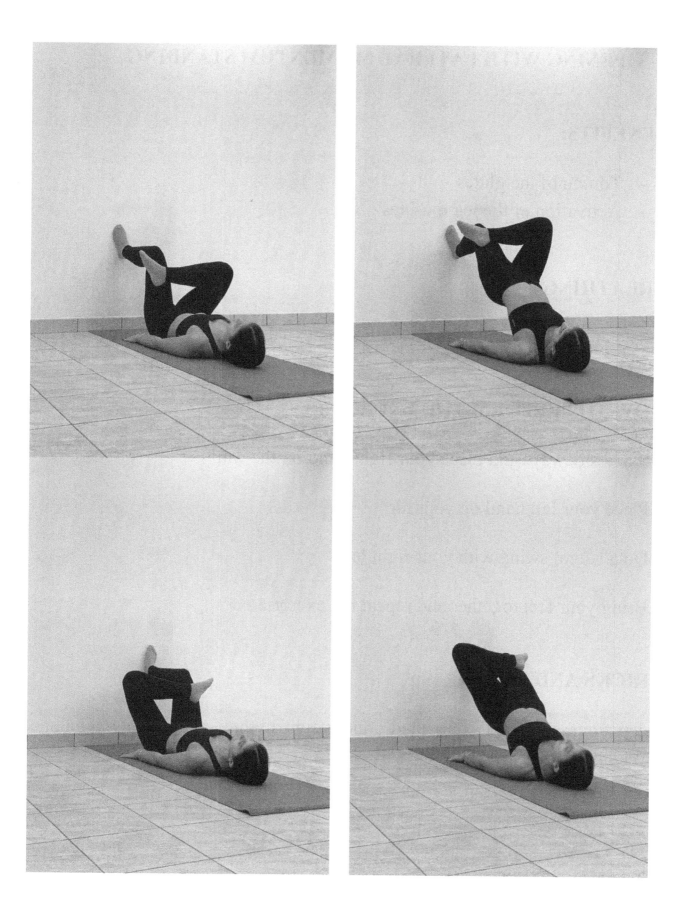

6 - OPENING WITH LATERAL MOMENTUM STANDING

BENEFITS:

- Toning of the glutes
- Activation of the leg muscles

BREATHING

Inhale at the beginning of the exercise and exhale as you straighten your leg.

HOW TO PERFORM THE EXERCISE

1 Stand sideways and place your right hand on the wall

2 Place your left hand on your hip

3 Do a lateral swing with your right leg

4 Bring your feet together and repeat the exercise

TRICKS AND TIPS

Keep your abdomen contracted, find your rhythm, and maintain balance throughout the movement.

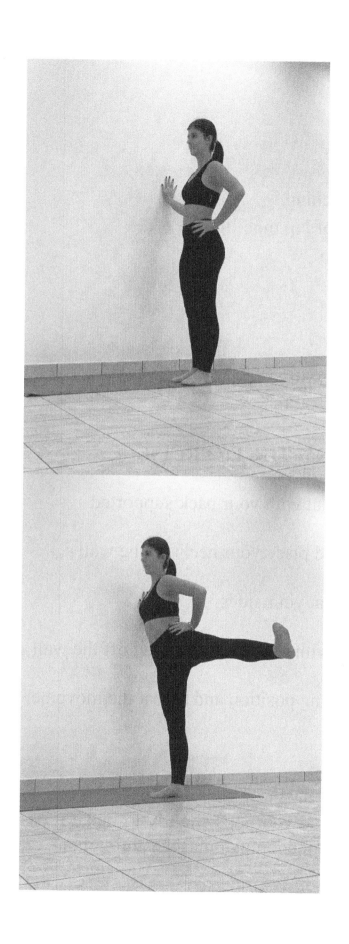

7 - SCISSORS

BENEFITS

- Adductor stretching
- Improvement of hip mobility
- Back relaxation

BREATHING

There is no particular rule to follow, maintain regular breathing.

HOW TO PERFORM THE EXERCISE

1 Lie down on the mat with your back supported

2 Raise your legs and place your heels on the wall

3 Extend your arms at your sides

4 Spread your legs without taking your feet off the wall

5 Return to the starting position and repeat the movement

TRICKS AND TIPS

At the beginning bend your legs slightly to make it easier to perform. Don't forget to engage your abdominal muscles throughout.

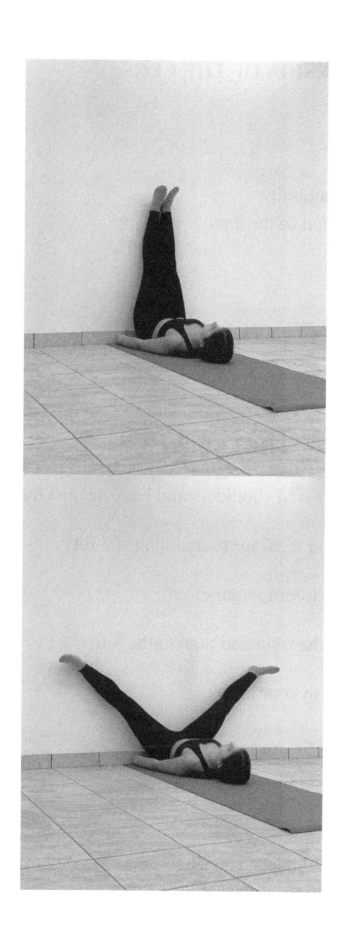

8 - DYNAMIC TORSION OF THE LEGS

BENEFITS:

- Improved hip mobility
- Dynamic rotation of the hips

BREATHING

Inhale when you are in the starting position and exhale when you move your knees.

HOW TO PERFORM THE EXERCISE

1 Sit on the mat with your shoulders and back against the wall

2 Place your hands on the floor to maintain stability

3 Bring your knees closer to your chest

4 Bend both legs to the right and then to the left

5 Touch the floor with your knees

6 Find your ideal pace

TRICKS AND TIPS

Do not force the stretching and concentrate on the abdomen which must remain contracted throughout the movement.

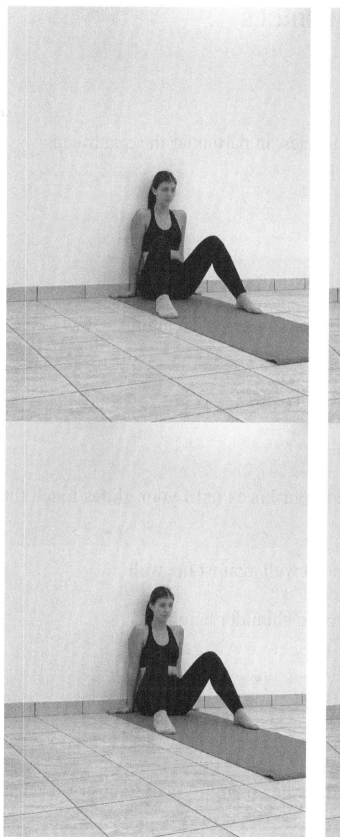
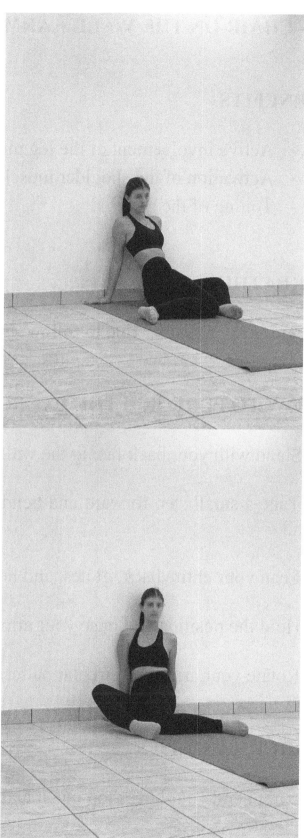

9 - CHAIR ON THE WALL + ARM CIRCLE

BENEFITS

- Active involvement of the leg muscles, in particular the quadriceps
- Activation of the shoulder muscles
- Toning of the glutes

BREATHING

There is no particular rule to follow, maintain regular breathing.

HOW TO PERFORM THE EXERCISE

1 Stand with your back facing the wall

2 Take a small step forward and bend your knees until your glutes touch the wall

3 Lean your entire back, glutes, and head well against the wall

4 Hold the position and raise your arms to shoulder height

5 Rotate your arms in a circular pattern

TRICKS AND TIPS

Do not bend your knees too much and create an angle equal to or greater than 90 degrees.

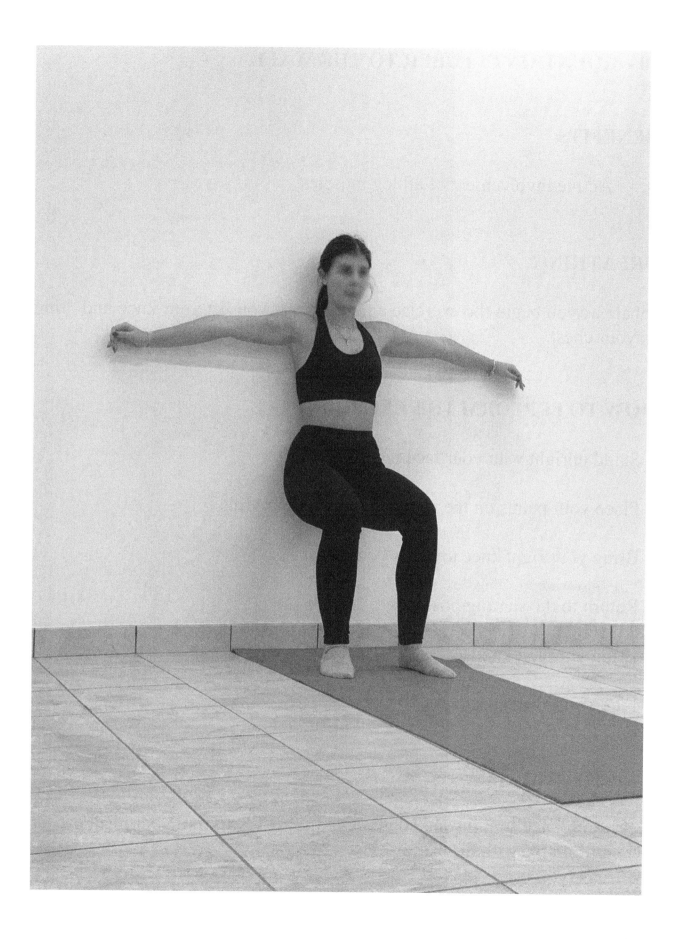

10 - MOUNTAIN CLIMBER TO THE WALL

BENEFITS

- Active involvement of all leg muscles

BREATHING

Inhale as you begin the exercise and exhale as you lift your knee and bring it to your chest.

HOW TO PERFORM THE EXERCISE

1 Stand upright with your face facing the wall

2 Place your palms on the wall and stretch your arms

3 Bring your right knee towards your chest

4 Return to the starting position

5 Bring your left knee towards your chest

6 Find your ideal pace

TRICKS AND TIPS

Keep your back straight and contract your abs. Try to find your ideal pace and get comfortable with the exercise.

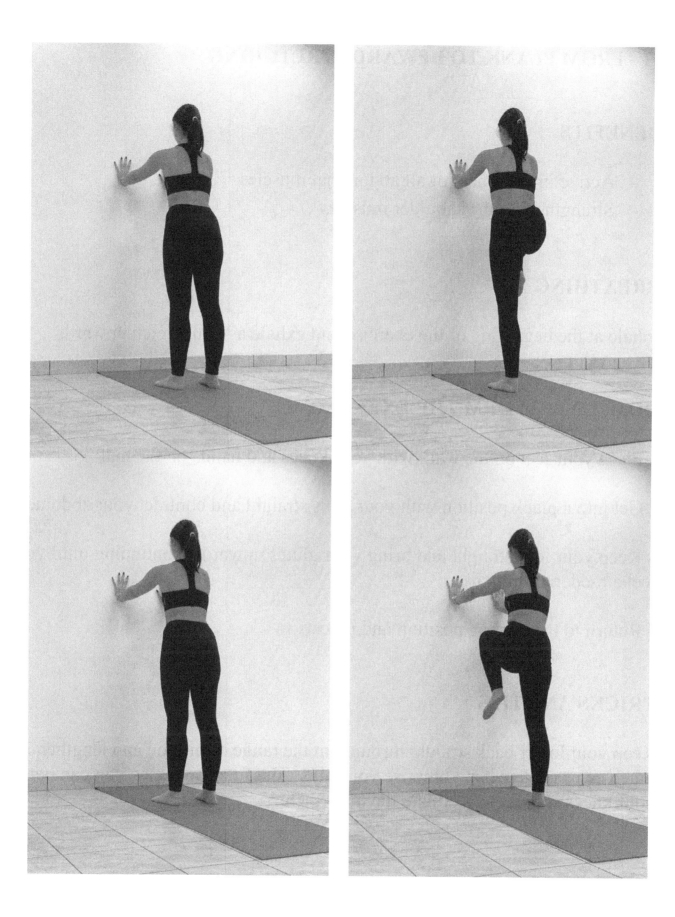

11 - FROM PLANK TO UPWARD STRETCHING

BENEFITS

- Active involvement of all abdominal muscles
- Strengthening the shoulder muscles

BREATHING

Inhale at the beginning of the exercise and exhale as you stretch upward.

HOW TO PERFORM THE EXERCISE

1 Place your feet on the wall, with your knees and hands on the mat

2 Get into a plank position with your arms straight and contract your abdomen

3 Keep your legs straight and bring your glutes upwards, continuing until you feel a moderate stretch

4 Return to the starting position and repeat

TRICKS AND TIPS

Keep your lower back straight throughout the range of motion and lengthen as much as possible when you raise your hips. The first few times you can bend your knees slightly to facilitate the movement.

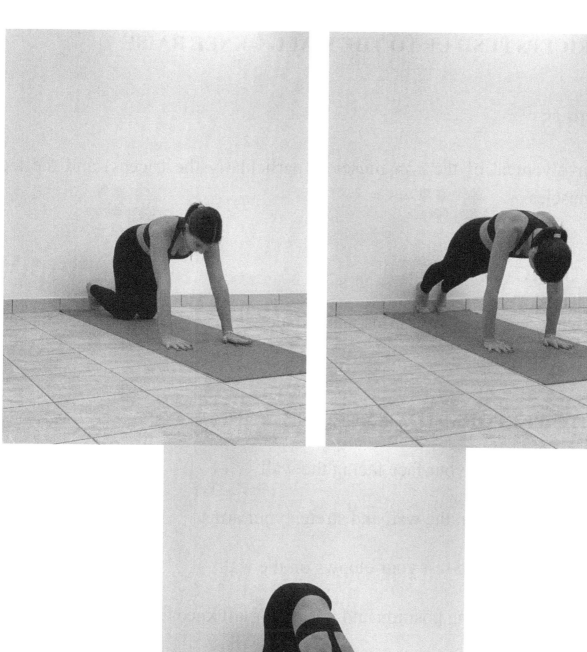
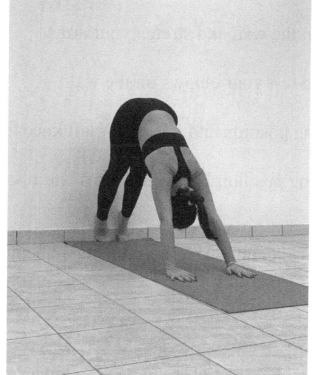

12 - TRICEPS PUSH UP TO THE WALL + KNEE RAISE

BENEFITS

- Involvement of the arm muscles (particularly the triceps) and the leg muscles

BREATHING

Inhale when you bend your arms and exhale when you return to the starting position.

HOW TO PERFORM THE EXERCISE

1 Stand upright with your face facing the wall

2 Place your palms on the wall and stretch your arms

3 Bend your arms and rest your elbows on the wall

4 Return to the starting position and raise your left knee towards your chest

5 Return to the starting position bend your arms and rest your elbows on the wall

6 Extend your arms again and repeat the same movement with the right leg

TRICKS AND TIPS

Keep your abdomen contracted and maintain your balance by focusing on your foot resting on the floor.

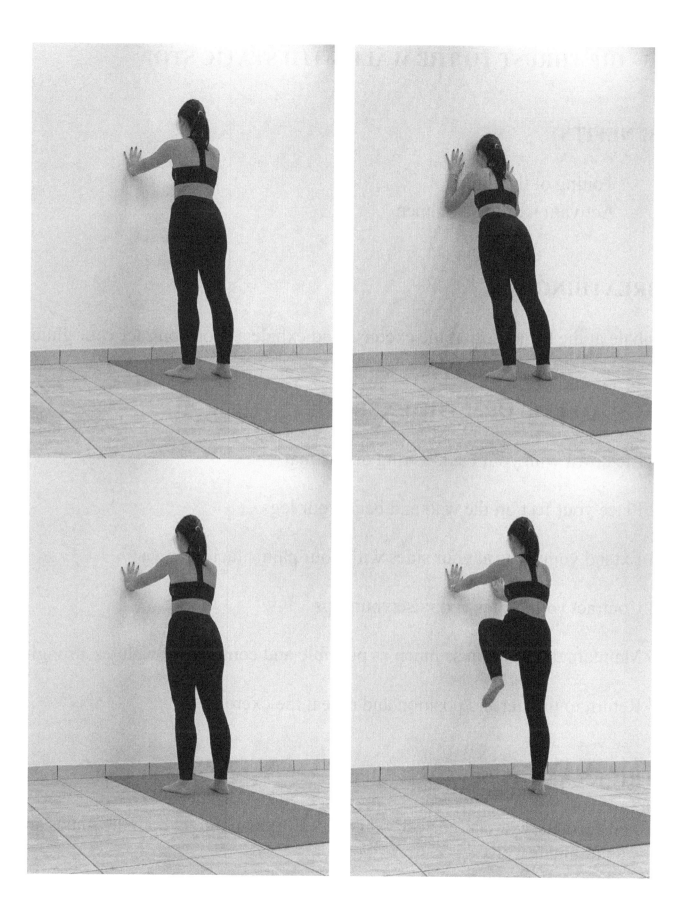

13 - HIP THRUST TO THE WALL WITH STATIC STOP

BENEFITS

- Toning of the glutes
- Activation of the abdomen

BREATHING

Inhale at the beginning of the exercise and exhale as you contract your glutes.

HOW TO PERFORM THE EXERCISE

1 Lie down with your back resting on the mat

2 Place your feet on the wall and bend your legs

3 Extend your arms at your sides with your palms facing down

4 Contract your glutes and raise your hips

5 Maintain the position as much as possible and contract your glutes strongly

6 Return to the starting position and repeat the exercise

TRICKS AND TIPS

To perform the exercise correctly it is necessary to contract both the glutes and the abdominals well.

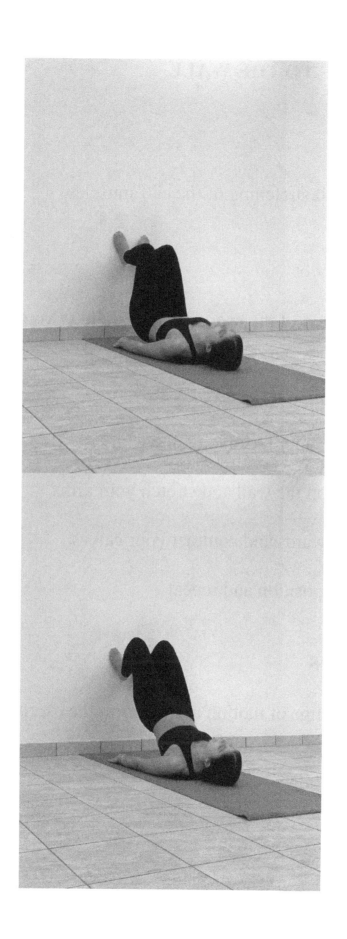

14 - CALF RAISES TO THE WALL

BENEFITS

- Stimulation and stretching of the calf muscles

BREATHING

Inhale at the beginning of the exercise and exhale as you raise your heels.

HOW TO PERFORM THE EXERCISE

1 Stand upright with your face facing the wall

2 Place your palms on the wall and stretch your arms

3 Lift your heels upwards and contract your calves

4 Return to starting position and repeat

TRICKS AND TIPS

Control the entire range of motion and perform the exercise slowly.

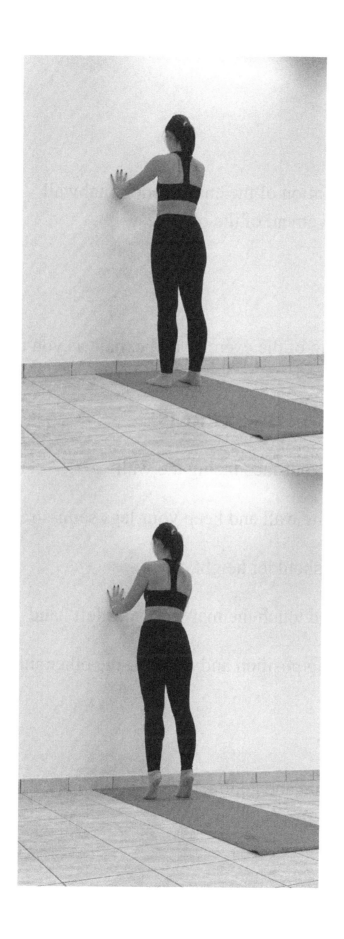

15 - RUSSIAN TWIST

BENEFITS

- Dynamic stimulation of the entire abdominal wall
- Particular involvement of the obliques

BREATHING

Inhale at the beginning of the exercise and exhale as you rotate.

HOW TO PERFORM THE EXERCISE

1 Sit on the mat with your face facing the wall

2 Place your feet on the wall and keep your legs semi-stretched

3 Raise your arms to shoulder height

4 Rotate to the left and touch the mat with your left hand

5 Return to the starting position and rotate to the other side

TRICKS AND TIPS

Keep your back straight and contract your abdominals. The execution must be slow and controlled.

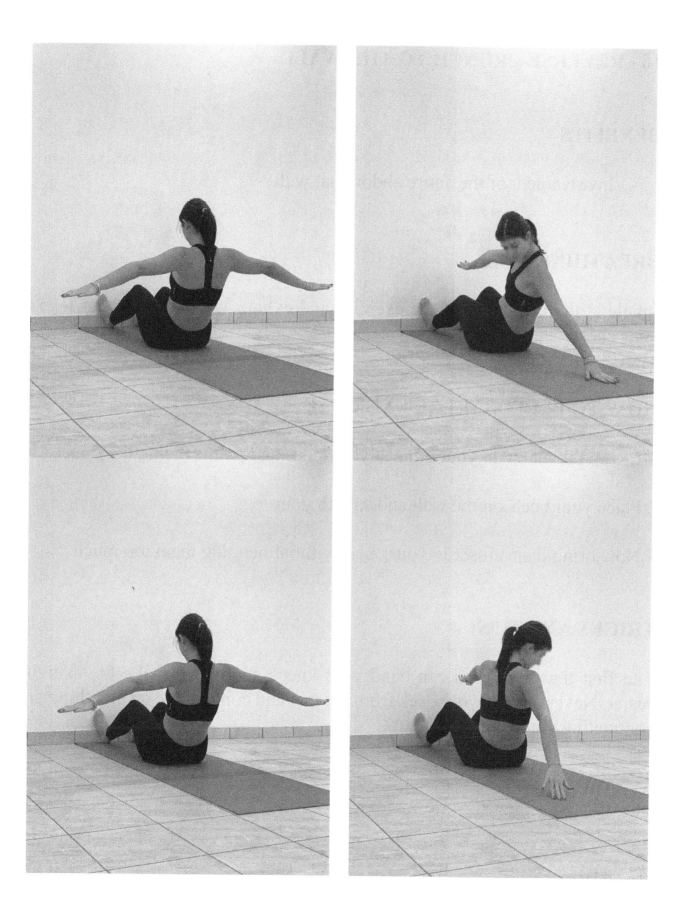

16 - REVERSE CRUNCH TO THE WALL

BENEFITS

- Involvement of the entire abdominal wall

BREATHING

Inhale at the beginning of the exercise and exhale as you bring your legs to your chest.

HOW TO PERFORM THE EXERCISE

1 Lie on the mat with your arms at your sides and palms facing the floor

2 Place your heels on the wall and stretch your legs

3 Now bring them closer to your chest without bending them too much

TRICKS AND TIPS

The first few times you can bend your knees slightly to make the exercise easier. Never remove your back from the mat and concentrate on breathing and contracting your abdomen.

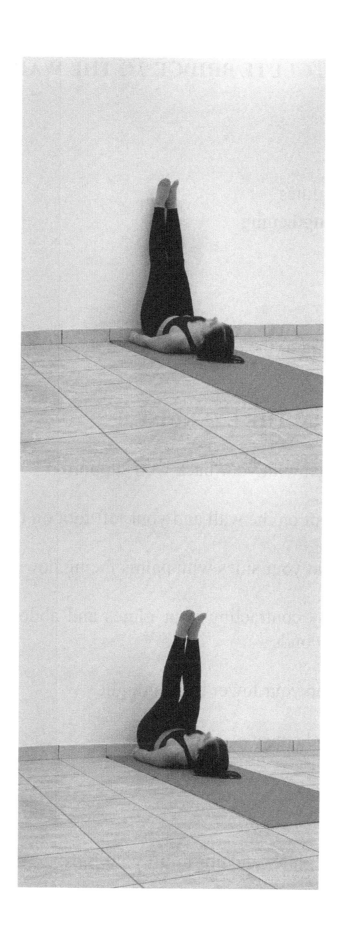

17 - UNILATERAL GLUTE BRIDGE TO THE WALL

BENEFITS

- Toning of the glutes
- Hamstring strengthening

BREATHING

Inhale at the beginning of the exercise and exhale as you raise your hips.

HOW TO PERFORM THE EXERCISE

1 Lie down on the mat with your back well supported

2 Place your right foot on the wall and your left foot on the mat

3 Extend your arms at your sides with palms facing down

4 Raise your hips by contracting your glutes and abdominals and hold the position for a few seconds

5 Make sure you keep your lower back straight

6 Descend slowly and repeat

TRICKS AND TIPS

Focus on using your glutes and abs to lift your hips.

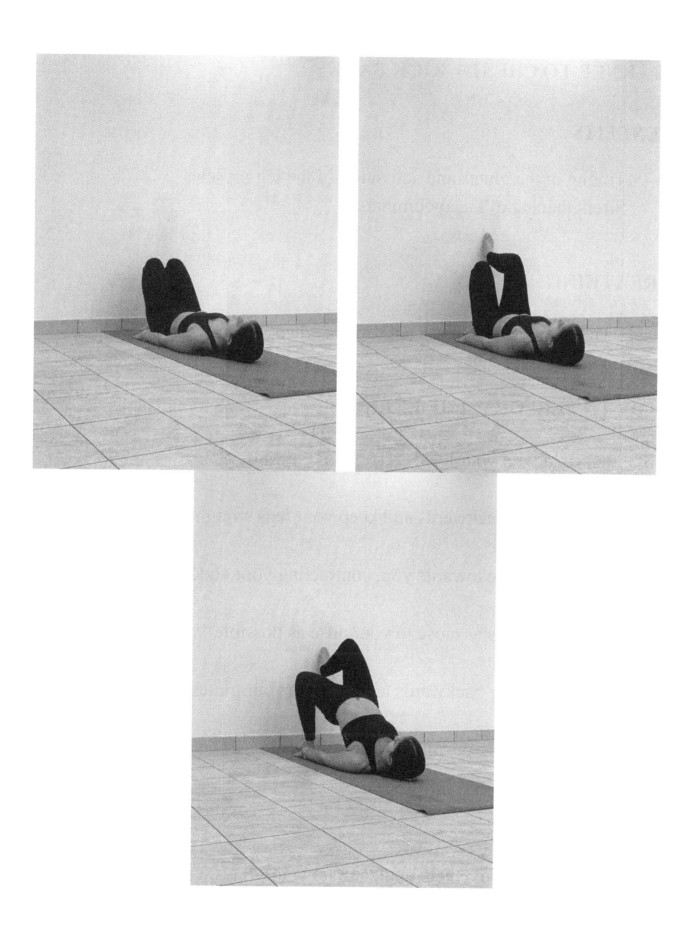

18 - KNEE TO CHEST + KICK BACK

BENEFITS

- Toning of the glutes and activation of the leg muscles
- Strengthening of the abdominals

BREATHING

Inhale when you lift your knee and exhale when you kick back.

HOW TO PERFORM THE EXERCISE

1 Stand upright with your hands resting on the wall

2 Take a small step backwards and keep your legs straight

3 Bring your left knee towards you, contracting your abdomen

4 Bring your left knee as close to your nose as possible

5 Extend your left leg backwards and contract your glutes

6 Return to the starting position and repeat the movement with the other leg

TRICKS AND TIPS

Concentrate on the movement and contract your glutes well when performing the kick-back.

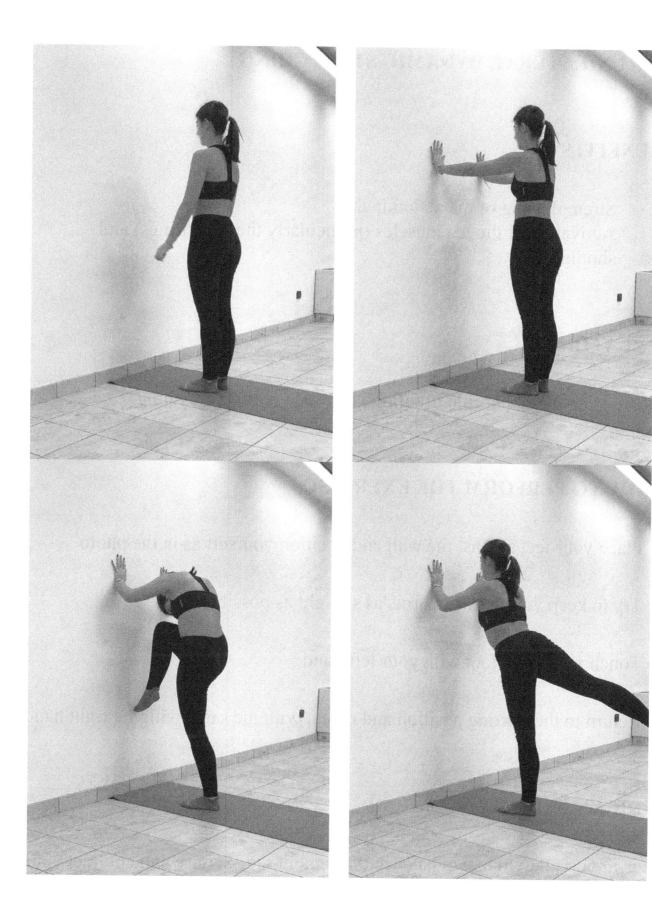

19 - UNILATERAL DYNAMIC STRETCHING

BENEFITS

- Strengthening of the abdominals
- Activation of the leg muscles (particularly the hamstrings) and shoulders

BREATHING

There is no particular rule to follow, maintain regular breathing.

HOW TO PERFORM THE EXERCISE

1 Place your feet against the wall and position yourself as in the photo

2 Try to keep your legs and arms as straight as possible

3 Touch your right foot with your left hand

4 Return to the starting position and repeat with the same with the right hand

TRICKS AND TIPS

It is important to maintain balance throughout the exercise and contract your abdominals to remain stable and perform the movement more easily.

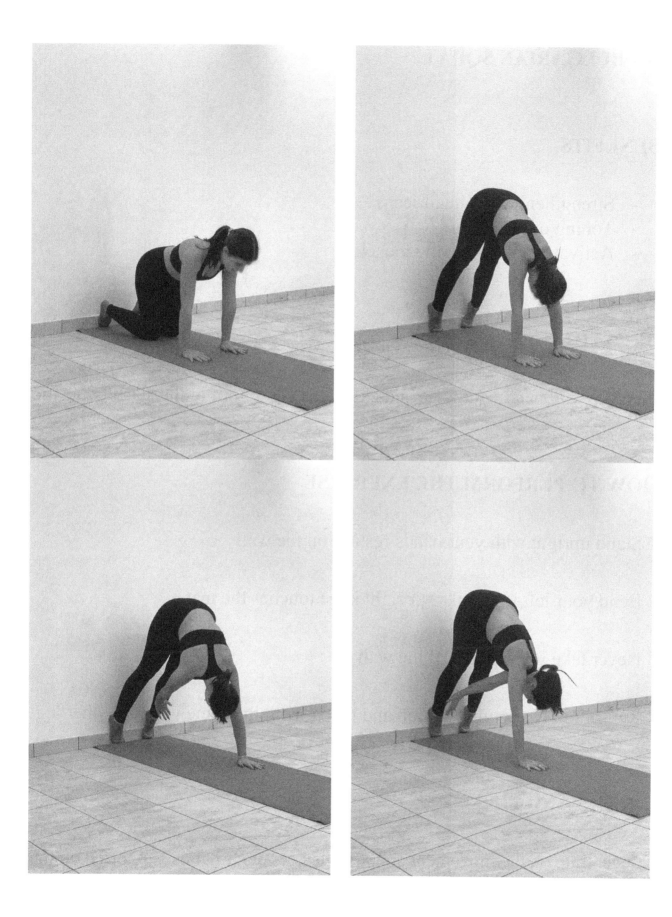

20 - BULGARIAN SQUAT

BENEFITS

- Strengthening the quadriceps
- Toning of the glutes
- Activation of stabilizing muscles

BREATHING

Inhale as you bend your knee and exhale as you return to the starting position.

HOW TO PERFORM THE EXERCISE

1 Stand upright with your hands resting on the wall

2 Bend your left leg until your right knee touches the mat

3 Never take your hands off the wall

4 Return to the starting position and repeat with the same with the other leg

TRICKS AND TIPS

Concentrate on the movement and always keep your hands supported on the wall to maintain stability throughout the entire execution range.

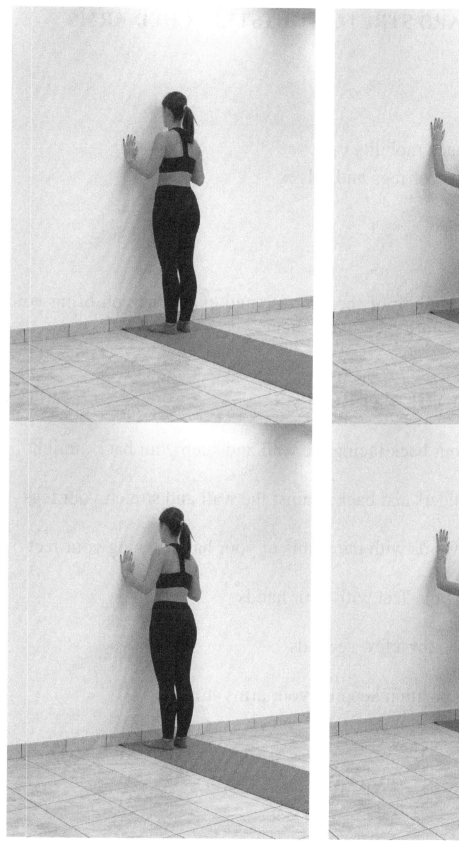
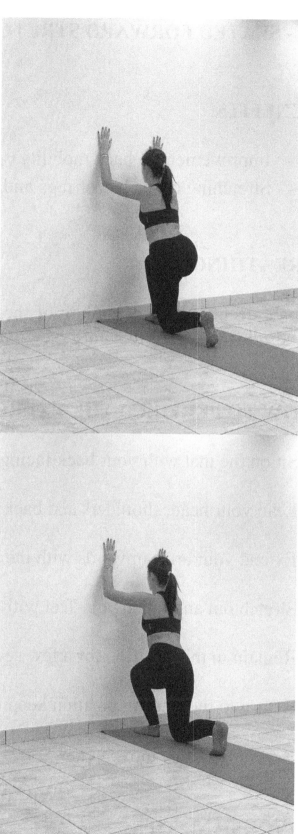

21 - SEATED FORWARD STRETCH-OUTSTRETCHED ARMS

BENEFITS:

- Improvement of back mobility
- Stretching of the hamstrings and calves

BREATHING:

Inhale deeply at the beginning of the exercise and exhale as you bring your hands closer to your feet until they touch them.

HOW TO PERFORM THE EXERCISE:

1 Sit on the mat with your back facing the wall and keep your back straight

2 Lean your head, shoulders and back against the wall and stretch your legs

3 Extend your arms upwards with the palms of your hands facing your feet

4 Stretch out and touch your feet with your hands

7 Remain in this position for a few seconds

8 Return to the starting position keeping your arms straight

9 Repeat the same movement

TRICKS AND TIPS:

Bend your legs slightly, this will help you touch your feet more easily.

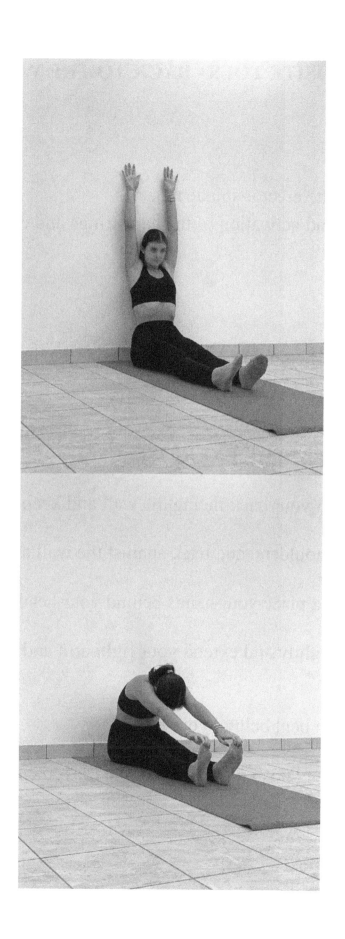

22 - TOUCH OPPOSITE TOES - BACK TO THE WALL

BENEFITS

- Stretching of the erector spinae muscles
- Involvement and activation of the hamstrings and calves

BREATHING

Inhale deeply at the beginning of the exercise and exhale as you bring your hand closer to your foot until it touches it.

HOW TO PERFORM THE EXERCISE

1 Sit on the mat with your back facing the wall and keep your back straight

2 Lean your head, shoulders, and back against the wall and stretch your legs

3 Fold your arms and place your hands behind your head

4 Open your legs slightly and extend your right arm and touch the toe of your left foot

5 Keep your left arm bent behind your head

6 Return to the starting position and repeat the movement with your left arm

TRICKS AND TIPS

Try to keep your legs straight without bending them excessively. Stretch your abs well when you bend.

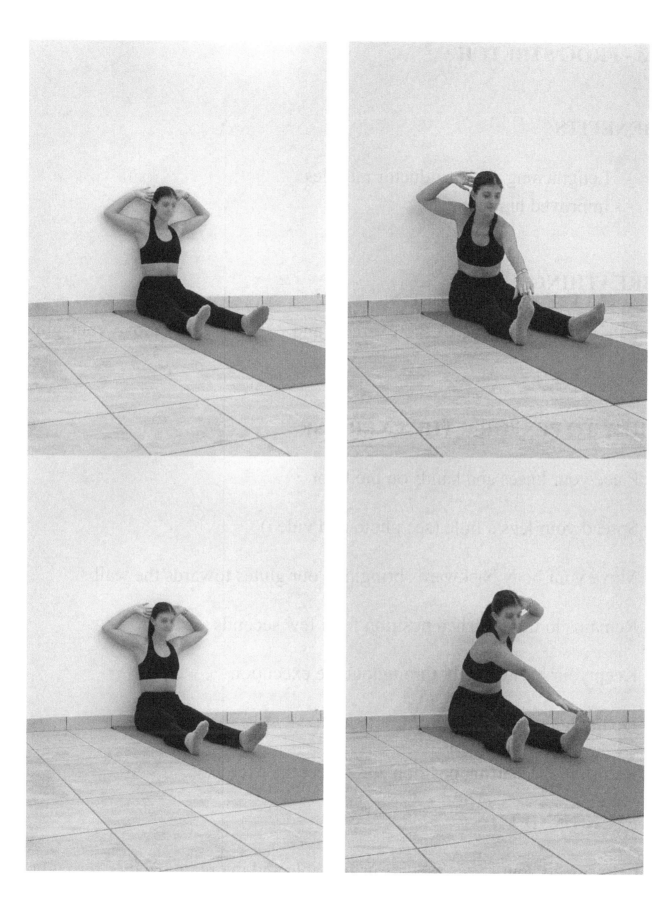

23 - FROG STRETCH

BENEFITS

- Lengthening of the adductor muscles
- Improved hip mobility

BREATHING

Inhale at the beginning of the exercise and exhale as you move your glutes back.

HOW TO PERFORM THE EXERCISE

1 Place your knees and hands on the floor

2 Spread your legs a little (see photo and video)

3 Move your body backwards bringing your glutes towards the wall

4 Remains in the stretched position for a few seconds

5 Keep your back straight throughout the execution

6 Do not take your hands off the floor

7 Return to the starting position and repeat the exercise

TRICKS AND TIPS

Try to spread your knees as wide as possible and maintain balance throughout the movement.

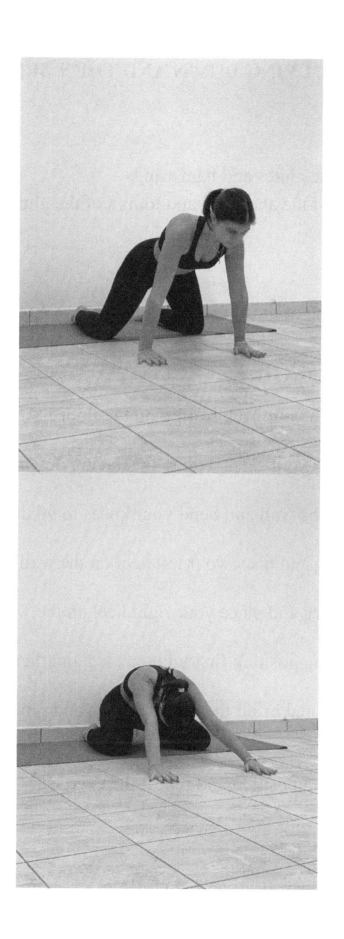

24 - WALK WHILE LYING DOWN AND THEN BRIDGE

BENEFITS

- Activation of the glutes and hamstrings
- Strengthening of the abdomen and toning of the glutes

BREATHING

Inhale at the beginning of the exercise and exhale as you raise your hips.

HOW TO PERFORM THE EXERCISE

1 Lie on the floor with your back resting on the floor

2 Extend your arms at your sides with palms facing down

3 Place your feet on the wall and bend your knees to 90 degrees

5 Extend your left leg and place your left heel on the wall

6 Extend your right leg and place your right heel on the wall

7 Return to the starting position first with one leg and then with the other

8 Activate the glutes and bring the hips upwards and remain in position for a few seconds

9 Return to the starting position and repeat the exercise

TRICKS AND TIPS

Do not curve your lower back and control the execution of the exercise by keeping your abdomen contracted.

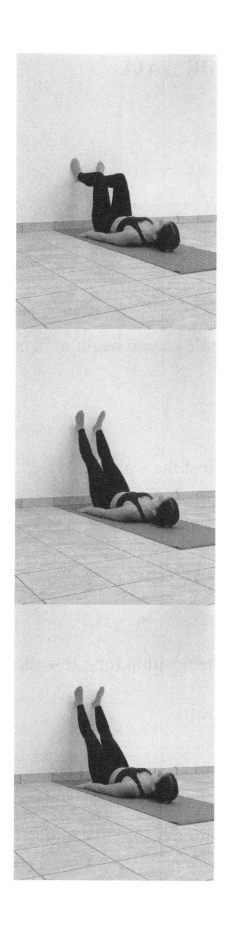
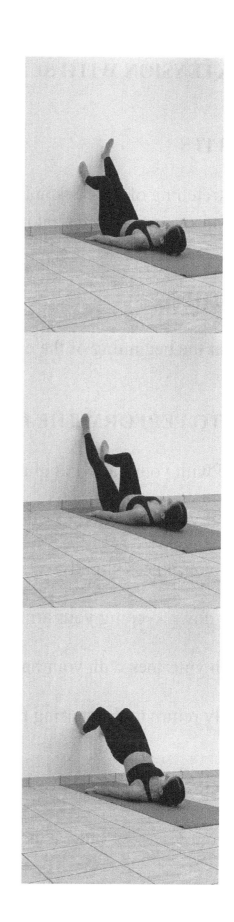

25 - EXTENSION WITH SUPPORT ON THE WALL

BENEFITS

- Stretching of the back and hamstrings
- Improvement of general mobility

BREATHING

Inhale at the beginning of the exercise and exhale as you begin to bend down.

HOW TO PERFORM THE EXERCISE

1 Stand with your back and glutes leaning against the wall

2 Extend your arms at your sides

3 Bend your knees slightly

4 Bend down keeping your arms relaxed

5 Touch your toes with your hands and hold the position for a few seconds

6 Slowly return to the starting position and repeat

TRICKS AND TIPS

Bend your knees as little as possible and do not detach your glutes from the wall.

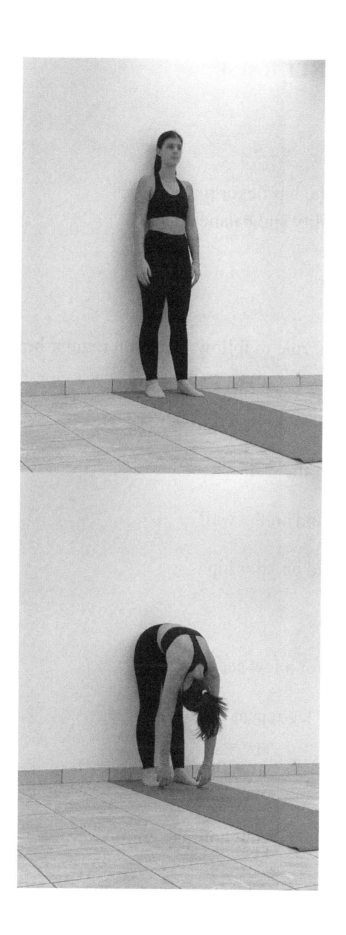

26 - STANDING KNEE RAISE

BENEFITS

- Activation of the hip flexor muscles
- Improved stability and balance

BREATHING

There is no particular rule to follow, maintain regular breathing.

HOW TO PERFORM THE EXERCISE:

1 Stand to the side of the wall

2 Place your right hand on the wall

3 Place your left hand on your hip

4 Raise your right knee

5 Hold the position for a few seconds

6 Slowly lower your leg repeat with the left leg

TRICKS AND TIPS

Keep your back straight throughout the entire exercise.

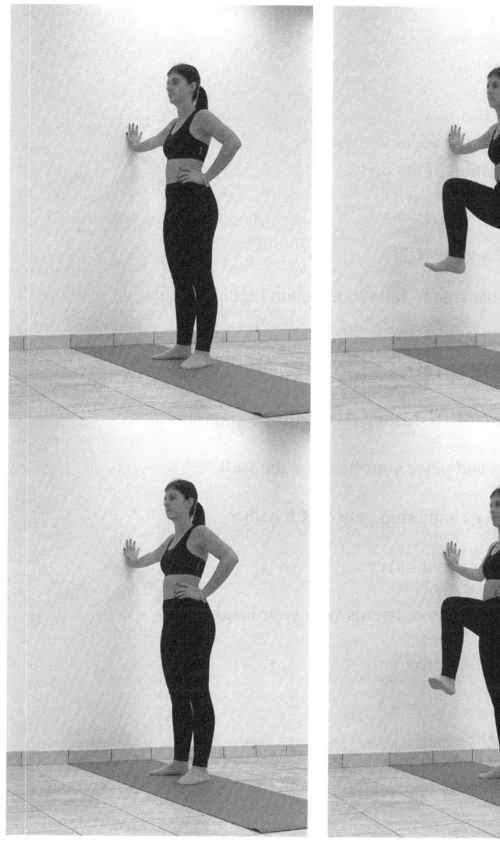
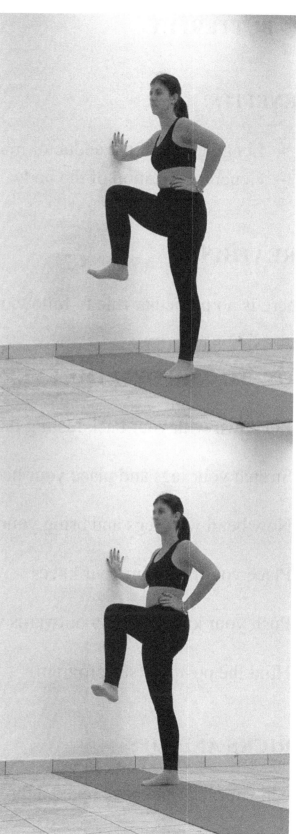

27 - BUTTERFLY

BENEFITS:

- Lengthening of the adductor muscles
- General relaxation of the body

BREATHING

There is no particular rule to follow, maintain regular breathing.

HOW TO PERFORM THE EXERCISE

1 Lie down with your back resting on the floor

2 Stretch your legs and place your heels on the wall

3 Now bend your legs and bring your feet together

4 Place your hands on your knees

5 Push your knees slightly outwards with your hands

6 Hold the position (see program)

TRICKS AND TIPS

Keep your legs and back relaxed throughout the execution.

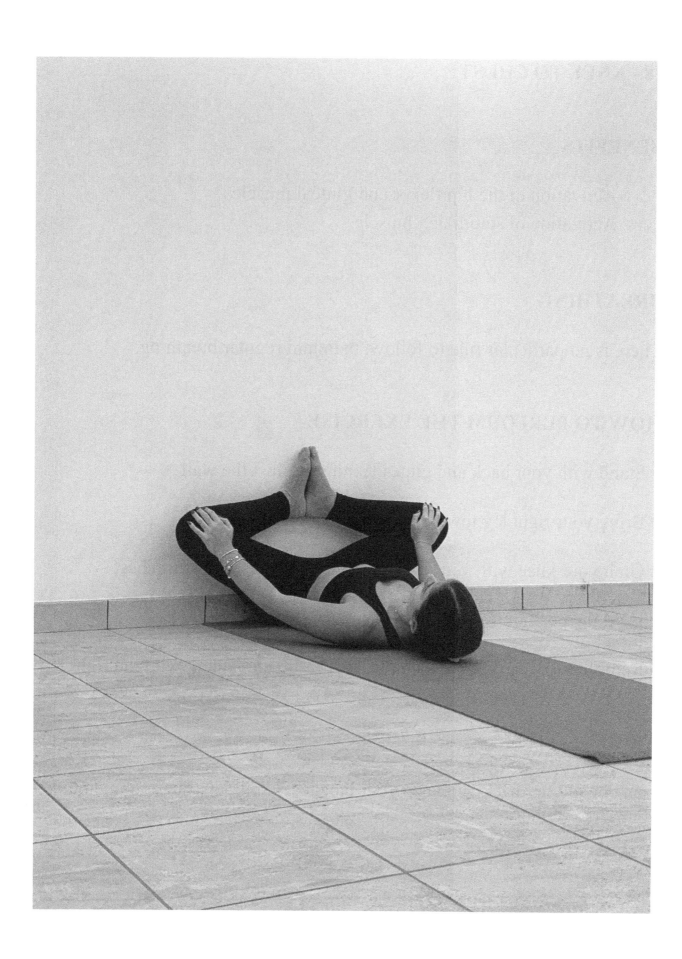

28 - KNEE TO CHEST

BENEFITS

- Activation of the hip flexor and gluteal muscles
- Activation of stabilizing muscles

BREATHING

There is no particular rule to follow, maintain regular breathing.

HOW TO PERFORM THE EXERCISE

1 Stand with your back and glutes leaning against the wall

2 Bring your right leg towards you by bending the knee

3 Grab your knee with your hands and bring it closer to your chest

4 Hold the position for 2-3 seconds

5 Return to the starting position and repeat the movement with the right leg

TRICKS AND TIPS

Don't bend your back and keep your balance. Contract your abdomen to keep your torso rigid.

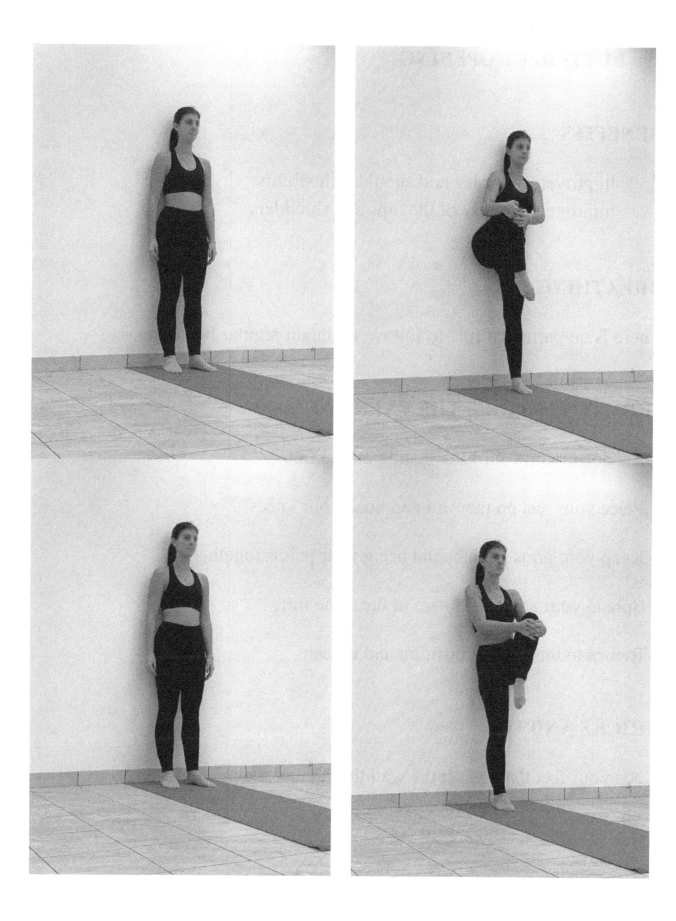

29 - BUTTERFLY OPENING

BENEFITS

- Improvement of leg and shoulder flexibility
- Improved mobility of the hips and shoulders

BREATHING

There is no particular rule to follow, maintain regular breathing.

HOW TO PERFORM THE EXERCISE

1 Lie down with your back resting on the floor

2 Place your feet on the wall and bend your knees

3 Keep your arms straight and bring your palms together

4 Spread your arms and knees at the same time

5 Return to the starting position and repeat

TRICKS AND TIPS

Keep your feet flat against the wall throughout the movement.

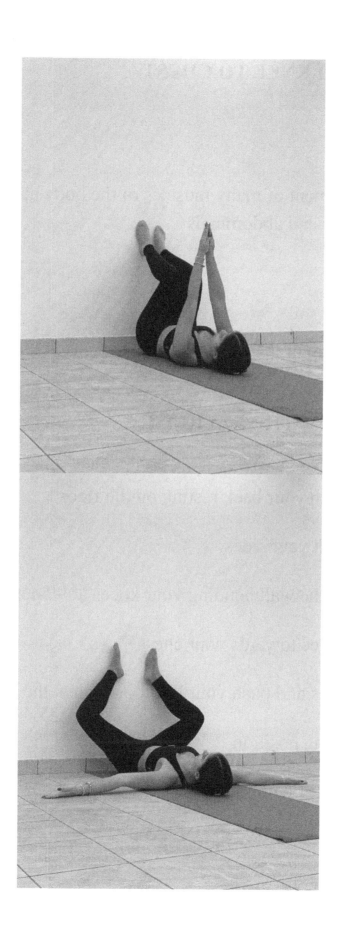

30 - BRIDGE WITH KNEE TO CHEST

BENEFITS

- Active involvement of many muscles of the body at the same time
- Focus on glutes and abdominals

BREATHING

Inhale at the beginning of the exercise and exhale as you contract your glutes.

HOW TO PERFORM THE EXERCISE

1 Lie on the floor with your back resting on the floor

2 Extend your arms at your sides

3 Place your feet on the wall bending your knees at 90 degrees

4 Bring your right knee towards your chest

5 Contract your glutes and push your left foot against the wall

6 Return to the starting position

7 Repeat the movement with the left leg

TRICKS AND TIPS

Contract your abs throughout the exercise to keep your back straight.

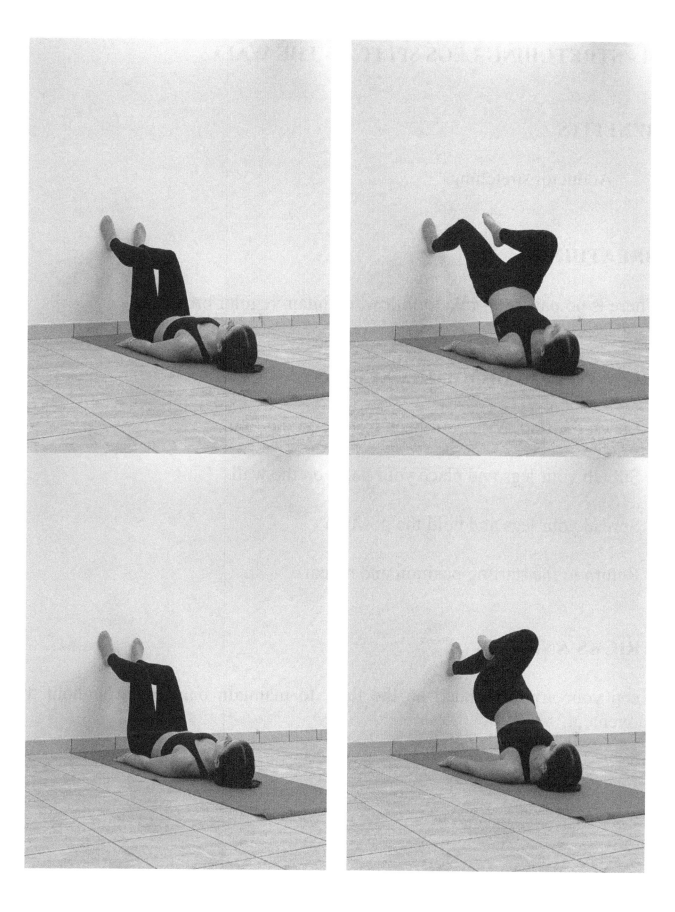

31 - STRETCHING LEGS SPLIT TO THE WALL

BENEFITS

- Adductor stretching

BREATHING

There is no particular rule to follow, maintain regular breathing.

HOW TO PERFORM THE EXERCISE

1 Lie on the floor with your back resting on the floor

2 Stretch your legs and place your heels on the wall

3 Spread your legs and hold the position

4 Return to the starting position and repeat

TRICKS AND TIPS

Keep your arms extended on the floor to maintain balance throughout the movement.

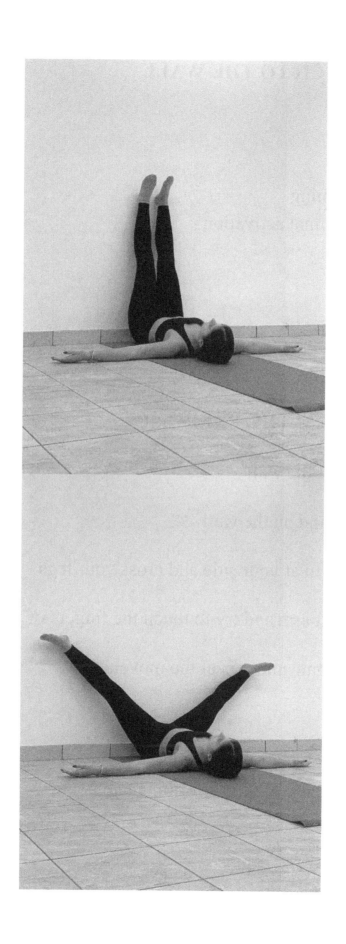

32 - BACK STRETCH TO THE WALL

BENEFITS

- Dorsal lengthening
- Oblique abdominal activation

BREATHING

Inhale in the starting position and exhale as you begin the movement.

HOW TO PERFORM THE EXERCISE

1 Stand to the side of the wall

2 Place your right hand on the wall

3 Extend your left arm at your side and cross your legs

4 Now raise your left arm and try to touch the fingers of your right hand

5 Lower your arm again and repeat the movement

TRICKS AND TIPS

Try not to bend your legs while performing and not take your feet off the floor.

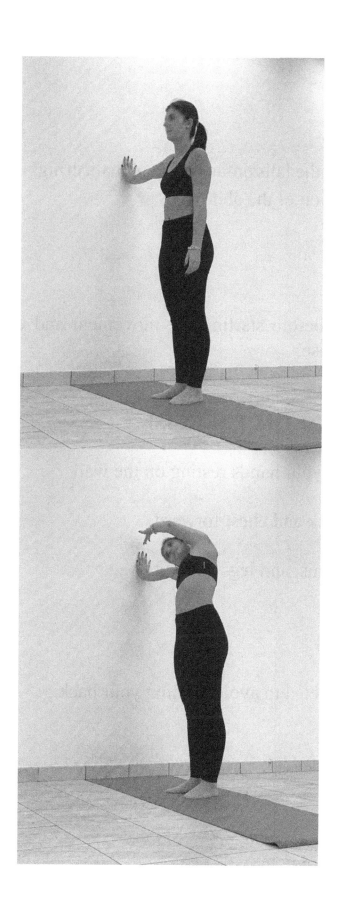

33 - DYNAMIC EXTENSION TO THE WALL

BENEFITS

- Lengthening of the latissimus dorsi and hamstrings
- Active contraction of the abdomen

BREATHING

Take a deep breath before starting the movement and exhale slowly while performing the exercise.

HOW TO PERFORM THE EXERCISE

1 Stand upright with your hands resting on the wall

2 Bring your hips back and chest forward

3 Keep your back, arms, and legs straight

TRICKS AND TIPS

Keep your abs contracted to avoid arching your back.

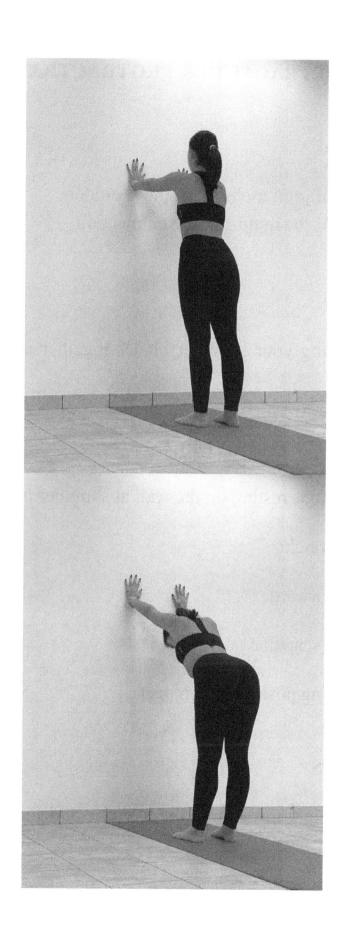

34 - SCAPULAR RETRACTION & PROTRACTION

BENEFITS

- Improvement of joint mobility of the shoulders
- Improvement of the mind-muscle connection

BREATHING

Inhale when you bring your shoulder blades together and exhale when you relax them.

HOW TO PERFORM THE EXERCISE

1 Stand with your hands resting on the wall at shoulder height

2 Keep your arms straight

3 Bring your chest forward

4 Start to adduct the scapulae

5 Return to the starting position and repeat

TRICKS AND TIPS

Keep your arms straight throughout the exercise and focus on your shoulder blades.

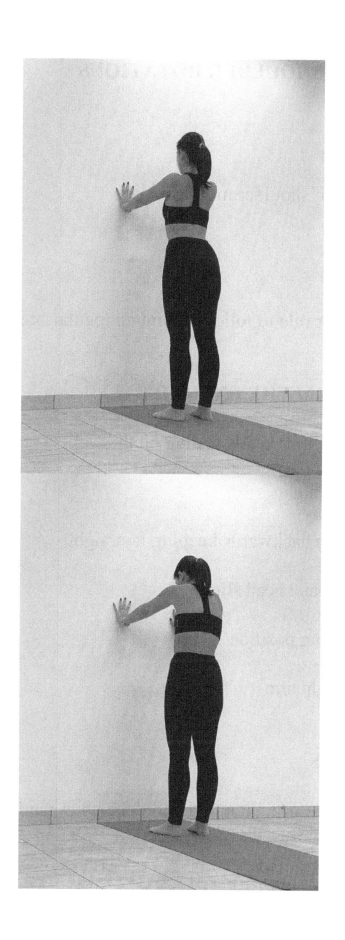

35 - ALTERNATE SHOULDER ROTATIONS

BENEFITS

- Improvement of shoulder mobility

BREATHING

There is no particular rule to follow, maintain regular breathing.

HOW TO PERFORM THE EXERCISE

1 Stand upright with your hands resting on the wall

2 Keep your arms straight

3 Bring your left arm backwards keeping it straight

4 Rotate your pelvis and head slightly

5 Return to the starting position

6 Repeat with the right arm

TRICKS AND TIPS

Try to keep your arms straight and do not take your hand off the wall.

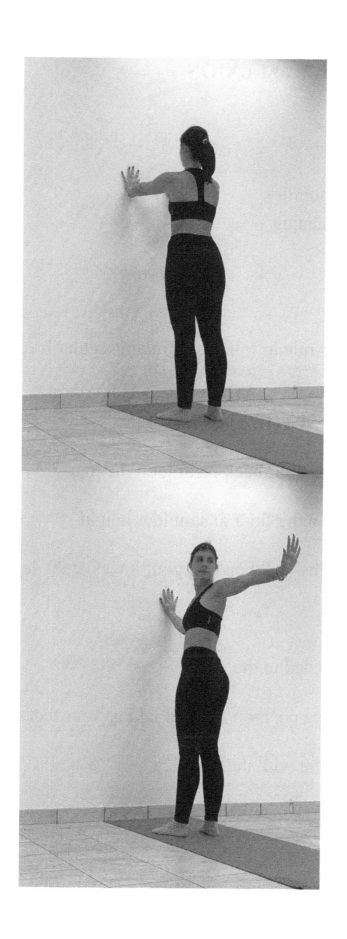

36 - ALTERNATE LEG FLEXION

BENEFITS

- Improved hip mobility
- Adductor lengthening

BREATHING

There is no particular rule to follow, maintain regular breathing.

HOW TO PERFORM THE EXERCISE

1 Lie on the floor with your back resting on the mat

2 Extend your arms on the floor at shoulder height

3 Place your feet on the wall bending your knees at 90 degrees

4 Spread your left leg

5 Keep both feet attached to the wall

6 Return to the starting position without taking your feet off the wall

7 Repeat the movement with the right leg

TRICKS AND TIPS

Keep your abs contracted during the movement and keep your back straight with the help of your arms.

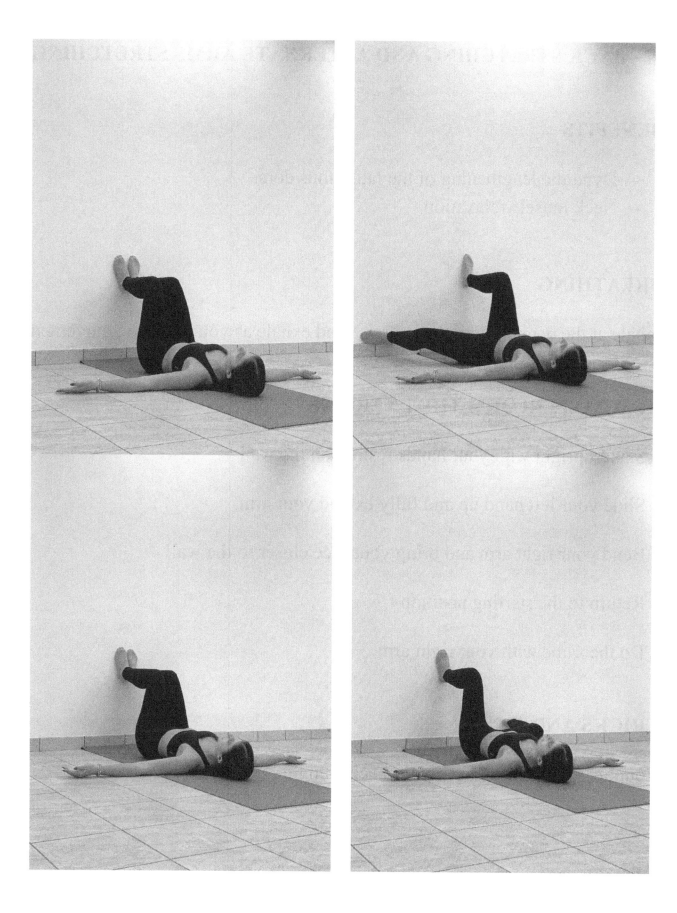

37 - BACK STRETCHING AND ALTERNATE ARMS STRETCHING

BENEFITS

- Dynamic lengthening of the latissimus dorsi
- Neck muscle relaxation

BREATHING

Inhale at the beginning of the exercise and exhale as you begin the movement.

HOW TO PERFORM THE EXERCISE

1 Stand upright with your hands resting on the wall

2 Slide your left hand up and fully extend your arm

3 Bend your right arm and bring your face closer to the wall

4 Return to the starting position

5 Do the same with your right arm

TRICKS AND TIPS

Contract your abs and keep your back straight.

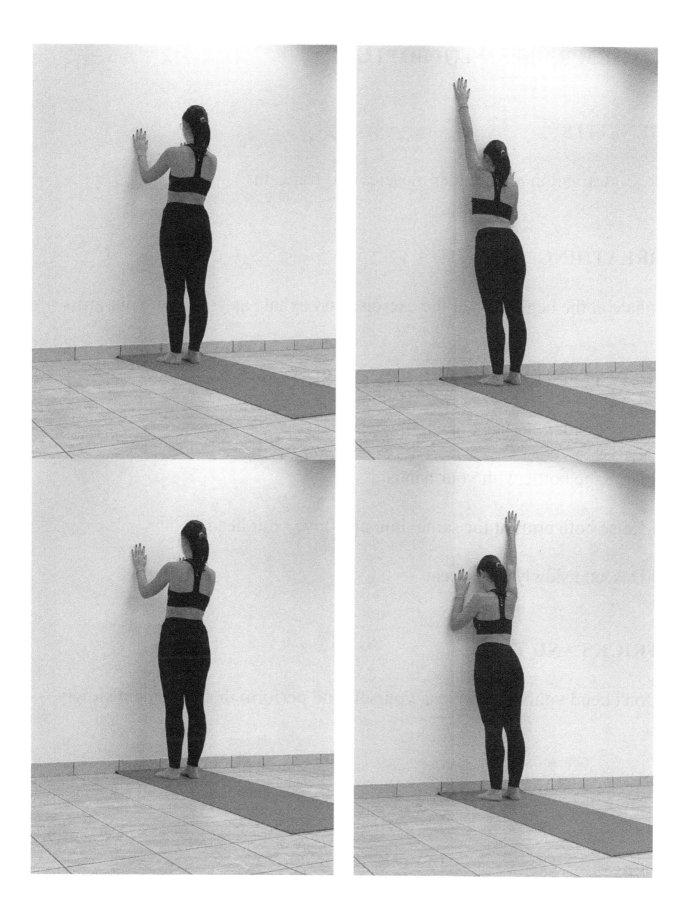

38 - ARM RAISES WITH BOTTLE

BENEFITS

- Activation of shoulder muscles and trapezius

BREATHING

Inhale at the beginning of the exercise and exhale as you raise your arms.

HOW TO PERFORM THE EXERCISE

1 Stand with your back facing the wall

2 Grab the bottle with your hands

3 Raise both arms at the same time up above your head

4 Descend slowly and repeat

TRICKS AND TIPS

Don't bend your back to push yourself and perform the movement slowly.

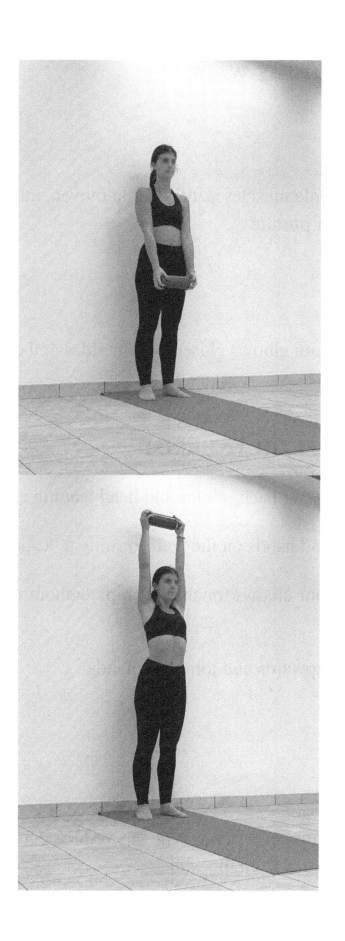

39 - PUSH BACK TO THE WALL

BENEFITS

- Involving multiple muscles with a single movement
- Improvement of posture

BREATHING

Inhale as you bring your elbows closer to your sides and exhale as you extend your arms upwards.

HOW TO PERFORM THE EXERCISE

1 Stand upright with your back, glutes and head leaning against the wall

2 Rest your elbows and hands on the wall forming a 90-degree angle

3 Push down until your elbows touch your hips without taking your arms off the wall

4 Extend your arms upwards and join your hands

5 Go down slowly

TRICKS AND TIPS

If you don't have enough experience, you can reduce the range of motion and slightly detach your arms from the wall.

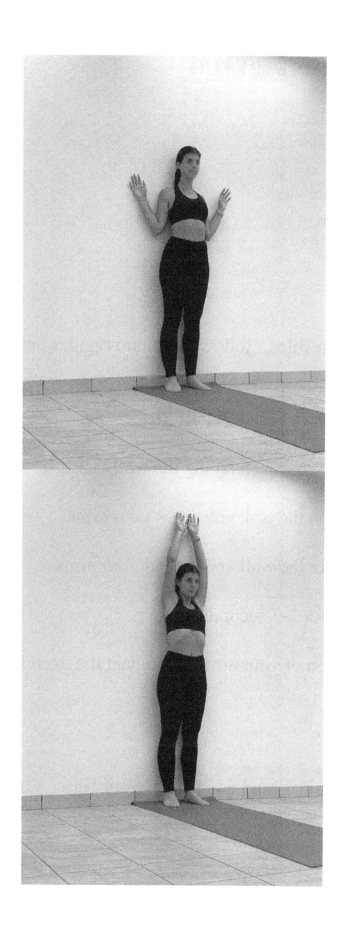

40 - CROSSED ARMS STRETCH

BENEFITS

- Stretching of the abs
- Back relaxation

BREATHING

There is no particular rule to follow, maintain regular breathing.

HOW TO PERFORM THE EXERCISE

1 Stand upright with your face facing the wall

2 Place your hands on the wall and cross your arms

3 Slide your palms on the wall and extend your arms

4 Hold the position for 2-3 seconds

5 Reverse the position of your arms and repeat the exercise

TRICKS AND TIPS

Contract your abdominals and don't curve your back.

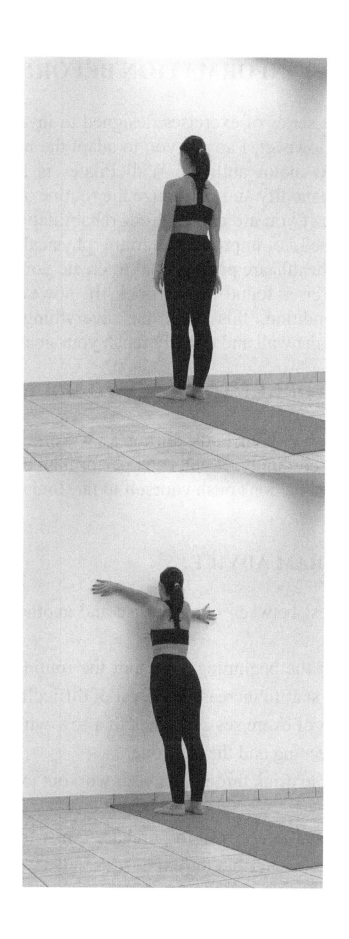

IMPORTANT INFORMATION BEFORE YOU START!

This book contains a series of exercises designed to involve all the muscular areas of your body, however, I advise you to adapt the movements according to your physical and motor abilities. Wall Pilates is highly customizable, therefore, feel free to modify and customize the routine based on your starting condition and needs. If you are carrying out rehabilitation activity due to an injury or if you need to improve a certain physical ability, follow the instructions of your healthcare professional to create your own routine with a selection of the exercises found in this book. If, however, you start from a normal physical condition, this book has everything you need to start practicing Pilates on the wall and quickly reach your goals.

DON'T FORGET TO LISTEN TO YOUR BODY!

It is essential to listen to your body during each workout and, if necessary, adapt your routine accordingly. If you can't perform an exercise correctly due to a physical impediment, don't push yourself to far, find a similar exercise and replace it.

TRAINING PROGRAM ADVICE:

- **Recovery times:** between one exercise and another, recover for 60-90 seconds.
- **Repetitions:** at the beginning carry out the routine only once, as time passes you can start to increase the level of difficulty by carrying out the same repetition of exercises 2-3 times in a row with a 2-3 minute break between one evening and the next one.
- **Hydration:** try to drink throughout your workout to keep your body well hydrated
- **Use of the mat:** I advise you to purchase a mat (standard yoga mat or similar) in order to carry out the exercises safely. Without a mat, you risk slipping and hurting yourself.
- **suitable clothing:** choose sporty and comfortable clothing

28-DAY FAT BURNING CHALLENGE

DAY 1

DATE: _____

NAME OF THE EXERCISE	EXERCISE	PAGE	REPETITIONS/ DURATION	✓
WALL SITTING POSITION	2	3	10-15 SECONDS	
UNILATERAL GLUTE BRIDGE TO THE WALL	17	33	5 REPETITIONS PER LEG	
TRICEPS PUSH UP TO THE WALL + KNEE RAISE	12	23	10 REPETITIONS	
KNEE TO CHEST	28	55	5 REPETITIONS PER LEG	
PUSH BACK TO THE WALL	39	77	10 REPETITIONS	

(The last column of the table is for you, use a pen to fill the cell every time you complete the exercise)

DAY 2

DATE: _____

NAME OF THE EXERCISE	EXERCISE	PAGE	REPETITIONS/ DURATION	✓
DYNAMIC EXTENSION TO THE WALL	33	65	10 REPETITIONS	
TORSION WITH SUPPORT	1	1	10 REPETITIONS PER SIDE	
BUTTERFLY OPENING	29	57	10 REPETITIONS	
BACK STRETCH TO THE WALL	32	63	10 REPETITIONS PER SIDE	
MOUNTAIN CLIMBER TO THE WALL	10	19	10 REPETITIONS PER LEG	

DAY 3

DATE: _____

NAME OF THE EXERCISE	EXERCISE	PAGE	REPETITIONS/ DURATION	✓
CHAIR ON THE WALL + ARM CIRCLE	9	17	10 REPETITIONS	
SINGLE LEG GLUTE BRIDGE	5	9	5 REPETITIONS PER SIDE	
CALF RAISES TO THE WALL	14	27	10 REPETITIONS	
SEATED FORWARD STRETCH- OUTSTRETCHED ARMS	21	41	10 REPETITIONS	
OPENING WITH LATERAL MOMENTUM STANDING	6	11	10 REPETITIONS PER LEG	

DAY 4

DATE: _____

NAME OF THE EXERCISE	EXERCISE	PAGE	REPETITIONS/ DURATION	✓
HIP FLEXOR STRETCHING	3	5	10 REPETITIONS PER LEG	
KNEE TO CHEST + KICK BACK	18	35	10 REPETITIONS PER LEG	
ALTERNATE LEG FLEXION	36	71	5 REPETITIONS PER LEG	
ARM RAISES WITH BOTTLE	38	75	10 REPETITIONS	
UNILATERAL DYNAMIC STRETCHING	19	37	5 REPETITIONS PER SIDE	

DAY 5

DATE: _____

NAME OF THE EXERCISE	EXERCISE	PAGE	REPETITIONS/ DURATION	✓
SCISSORS	7	13	10 REPETITIONS	
REVERSE CRUNCH TO THE WALL	16	31	10 REPETITIONS	
UNILATERAL GLUTE BRIDGE TO THE WALL	17	33	5 REPETITIONS PER LEG	
BUTTERFLY	27	53	30 SECONDS	
BUTTERFLY OPENING	29	57	10 REPETITIONS	

DAY 6

DATE: _____

NAME OF THE EXERCISE	EXERCISE	PAGE	REPETITIONS/ DURATION	✓
FROM PLANK TO UPWARD STRETCHING	11	21	5 REPETITIONS	
WALL SQUAT + KICK BACK	4	7	10 REPETITIONS	
TOUCH OPPOSITE TOES - BACK TO THE WALL	22	43	10 REPETITIONS PER SIDE	
STANDING KNEE RAISE	26	51	10 REPETITIONS PER LEG	
STRETCHING LEGS SPLIT TO THE WALL	31	61	10 REPETITIONS	

DAY 7

DATE: _____

NAME OF THE EXERCISE	EXERCISE	PAGE	REPETITIONS/ DURATION	✓
RUSSIAN TWIST	15	29	10 REPETITIONS PER SIDE	
EXTENSION WITH SUPPORT ON THE WALL	25	49	10 REPETITIONS	
BACK STRETCHING AND ALTERNATE ARMS	37	73	10 REPETITIONS PER SIDE	
DYNAMIC TORSION OF THE LEGS.	8	15	10 REPETITIONS PER SIDE	
CROSSED ARMS STRETCH	40	79	10 REPETITIONS	

DAY 8

DATE: _____

NAME OF THE EXERCISE	EXERCISE	PAGE	REPETITIONS/ DURATION	✓
FROG STRETCH	23	45	10 REPETITIONS	
WALK WHILE LYING DOWN AND THEN BRIDGE	24	47	5 REPETITIONS PER LEG	
ARM RAISES WITH BOTTLE	38	75	10 REPETITIONS	
HIP THRUST TO THE WALL WITH STATIC STOP	13	25	5 REPETITIONS	
ALTERNATE SHOULDER ROTATIONS	35	69	10 REPETITIONS PER SIDE	

DAY 9

DATE: _____

NAME OF THE EXERCISE	EXERCISE	PAGE	REPETITIONS/ DURATION	✓
TORSION WITH SUPPORT	1	1	10 REPETITIONS PER SIDE	
STRETCHING LEGS SPLIT TO THE WALL	31	61	10 REPETITIONS	
CROSSED ARMS STRETCH	40	79	10 REPETITIONS	
KNEE TO CHEST	28	55	5 REPETITIONS PER LEG	
WALL SITTING POSITION	2	3	10-15 SECONDS	

DAY 10

DATE: _____

NAME OF THE EXERCISE	EXERCISE	PAGE	REPETITIONS/ DURATION	✓
DYNAMIC EXTENSION TO THE WALL	33	65	10 REPETITIONS	
SEATED FORWARD STRETCH-OUTSTRETCHED ARMS	21	41	10 REPETITIONS	
ARM RAISES WITH BOTTLE	38	75	10 REPETITIONS	
UNILATERAL DYNAMIC STRETCHING	19	37	5 REPETITIONS PER SIDE	
BACK STRETCH TO THE WALL	32	63	10 REPETITIONS PER SIDE	

DAY 11

DATE: _____

NAME OF THE EXERCISE	EXERCISE	PAGE	REPETITIONS/ DURATION	✓
SCAPULAR RETRACTION & PROTRACTION	34	67	10 REPETITIONS	
UNILATERAL GLUTE BRIDGE TO THE WALL	17	33	5 REPETITIONS PER LEG	
TRICEPS PUSH UP TO THE WALL + KNEE RAISE	12	23	10 REPETITIONS	
REVERSE CRUNCH TO THE WALL	16	31	10 REPETITIONS	
BULGARIAN SQUAT	20	39	5 REPETITIONS PER LEG	

DAY 12

DATE: _____

NAME OF THE EXERCISE	EXERCISE	PAGE	REPETITIONS/ DURATION	✓
BUTTERFLY OPENING	29	57	10 REPETITIONS	
ALTERNATE LEG FLEXION	36	71	5 REPETITIONS PER LEG	
CHAIR ON THE WALL + ARM CIRCLE	9	17	10 REPETITIONS	
STANDING KNEE RAISE	26	51	10 REPETITIONS PER LEG	
PUSH BACK TO THE WALL	39	77	10 REPETITIONS	

DAY 13

DATE: _____

NAME OF THE EXERCISE	EXERCISE	PAGE	REPETITIONS/ DURATION	✓
WALK WHILE LYING DOWN AND THEN BRIDGE	24	47	5 REPETITIONS PER LEG	
FROM PLANK TO UPWARD STRETCHING	11	21	5 REPETITIONS	
BACK STRETCH TO THE WALL	32	63	10 REPETITIONS PER SIDE	
WALL SQUAT + KICK BACK	4	7	10 REPETITIONS	
HIP FLEXOR STRETCHING	3	5	10 REPETITIONS PER LEG	

DAY 14

DATE: _____

NAME OF THE EXERCISE	EXERCISE	PAGE	REPETITIONS/ DURATION	✓
BUTTERFLY	27	53	30 SECONDS	
KNEE TO CHEST + KICK BACK	18	35	10 REPETITIONS PER LEG	
EXTENSION WITH SUPPORT ON THE WALL	25	49	10 REPETITIONS	
CROSSED ARMS STRETCH	40	79	10 REPETITIONS	
SINGLE LEG GLUTE BRIDGE	5	9	5 REPETITIONS PER SIDE	

DAY 15

DATE: _____

NAME OF THE EXERCISE	EXERCISE	PAGE	REPETITIONS/ DURATION	✓
MOUNTAIN CLIMBER TO THE WALL	10	19	10 REPETITIONS PER LEG	
RUSSIAN TWIST	15	29	10 REPETITIONS PER SIDE	
OPENING WITH LATERAL MOMENTUM STANDING	6	11	10 REPETITIONS PER LEG	
TOUCH OPPOSITE TOES - BACK TO THE WALL	22	43	10 REPETITIONS PER SIDE	
STRETCHING LEGS SPLIT TO THE WALL	31	61	10 REPETITIONS	

DAY 16

DATE: _____

NAME OF THE EXERCISE	EXERCISE	PAGE	REPETITIONS/ DURATION	✓
SCISSORS	7	13	10 REPETITIONS	
DYNAMIC TORSION OF THE LEGS.	8	15	10 REPETITIONS PER SIDE	
UNILATERAL GLUTE BRIDGE TO THE WALL	17	33	5 REPETITIONS PER LEG	
CHAIR ON THE WALL + ARM CIRCLE	9	17	10 REPETITIONS	
CROSSED ARMS STRETCH	40	79	10 REPETITIONS	

DAY 17

DATE: _____

NAME OF THE EXERCISE	EXERCISE	PAGE	REPETITIONS/ DURATION	✓
BACK STRETCH TO THE WALL	32	63	10 REPETITIONS PER SIDE	
ALTERNATE SHOULDER ROTATIONS	35	69	10 REPETITIONS PER SIDE	
ARM RAISES WITH BOTTLE	38	75	10 REPETITIONS	
PUSH BACK TO THE WALL	39	77	10 REPETITIONS	
STANDING KNEE RAISE	26	51	10 REPETITIONS PER LEG	

DAY 18

DATE: _____

NAME OF THE EXERCISE	EXERCISE	PAGE	REPETITIONS/ DURATION	✓
BUTTERFLY OPENING	29	57	10 REPETITIONS	
UNILATERAL DYNAMIC STRETCHING	19	37	5 REPETITIONS PER SIDE	
BACK STRETCHING AND ALTERNATE ARMS	37	73	10 REPETITIONS PER SIDE	
TORSION WITH SUPPORT	1	1	10 REPETITIONS PER SIDE	
KNEE TO CHEST + KICK BACK	18	35	10 REPETITIONS PER LEG	

DAY 19

DATE: _____

NAME OF THE EXERCISE	EXERCISE	PAGE	REPETITIONS/ DURATION	✓
DYNAMIC EXTENSION TO THE WALL	33	65	10 REPETITIONS	
WALL SITTING POSITION	2	3	10-15 SECONDS	
FROG STRETCH	23	45	10 REPETITIONS	
WALK WHILE LYING DOWN AND THEN BRIDGE	24	47	5 REPETITIONS PER LEG	
EXTENSION WITH SUPPORT ON THE WALL	25	49	10 REPETITIONS	

DAY 20

DATE: _____

NAME OF THE EXERCISE	EXERCISE	PAGE	REPETITIONS/ DURATION	✓
MOUNTAIN CLIMBER TO THE WALL	10	19	10 REPETITIONS PER LEG	
RUSSIAN TWIST	15	29	10 REPETITIONS PER SIDE	
TOUCH OPPOSITE TOES - BACK TO THE WALL	22	43	10 REPETITIONS PER SIDE	
SEATED FORWARD STRETCH- OUTSTRETCHED ARMS	21	41	10 REPETITIONS	
HIP THRUST TO THE WALL WITH STATIC STOP	13	25	5 REPETITIONS	

DAY 21

DATE: _____

NAME OF THE EXERCISE	EXERCISE	PAGE	REPETITIONS/ DURATION	✓
KNEE TO CHEST	28	55	5 REPETITIONS PER LEG	
BUTTERFLY	27	53	30 SECONDS	
UNILATERAL GLUTE BRIDGE TO THE WALL	17	33	5 REPETITIONS PER LEG	
STANDING KNEE RAISE	26	51	10 REPETITIONS PER LEG	
REVERSE CRUNCH TO THE WALL	16	31	10 REPETITIONS	

DAY 22

DATE: _____

NAME OF THE EXERCISE	EXERCISE	PAGE	REPETITIONS/ DURATION	✓
SCISSORS	7	13	10 REPETITIONS	
CROSSED ARMS STRETCH	40	79	10 REPETITIONS	
WALL SQUAT + KICK BACK	4	7	10 REPETITIONS	
ALTERNATE LEG FLEXION	36	71	5 REPETITIONS PER LEG	
UNILATERAL DYNAMIC STRETCHING	19	37	5 REPETITIONS PER SIDE	

DAY 23

DATE: _____

NAME OF THE EXERCISE	EXERCISE	PAGE	REPETITIONS/ DURATION	✓
ARM RAISES WITH BOTTLE	38	75	10 REPETITIONS	
DYNAMIC TORSION OF THE LEGS.	8	15	10 REPETITIONS PER SIDE	
BACK STRETCH TO THE WALL	32	63	10 REPETITIONS PER SIDE	
PUSH BACK TO THE WALL	39	77	10 REPETITIONS	
FROM PLANK TO UPWARD STRETCHING	11	21	5 REPETITIONS	

DAY 24

DATE: _____

NAME OF THE EXERCISE	EXERCISE	PAGE	REPETITIONS/ DURATION	✓
BUTTERFLY OPENING	29	57	10 REPETITIONS	
CROSSED ARMS STRETCH	40	79	10 REPETITIONS	
HIP FLEXOR STRETCHING	3	5	10 REPETITIONS PER LEG	
SINGLE LEG GLUTE BRIDGE	5	9	5 REPETITIONS PER SIDE	
KNEE TO CHEST + KICK BACK	18	35	10 REPETITIONS PER LEG	

DAY 25

DATE: _____

NAME OF THE EXERCISE	EXERCISE	PAGE	REPETITIONS/ DURATION	✓
RUSSIAN TWIST	15	29	10 REPETITIONS PER SIDE	
EXTENSION WITH SUPPORT ON THE WALL	25	49	10 REPETITIONS	
ALTERNATE SHOULDER ROTATIONS	35	69	10 REPETITIONS PER SIDE	
OPENING WITH LATERAL MOMENTUM STANDING	6	11	10 REPETITIONS PER LEG	
WALL SITTING POSITION	2	3	10-15 SECONDS	

DAY 26

DATE: _____

NAME OF THE EXERCISE	EXERCISE	PAGE	REPETITIONS/ DURATION	✓
UNILATERAL DYNAMIC STRETCHING	19	37	5 REPETITIONS PER SIDE	
REVERSE CRUNCH TO THE WALL	16	31	10 REPETITIONS	
STRETCHING LEGS SPLIT TO THE WALL	31	61	10 REPETITIONS	
FROM PLANK TO UPWARD STRETCHING	11	21	5 REPETITIONS	
UNILATERAL GLUTE BRIDGE TO THE WALL	17	33	5 REPETITIONS PER LEG	

DAY 27

DATE: _____

NAME OF THE EXERCISE	EXERCISE	PAGE	REPETITIONS/ DURATION	✓
ALTERNATE LEG FLEXION	36	71	5 REPETITIONS PER LEG	
ARM RAISES WITH BOTTLE	38	75	10 REPETITIONS	
STANDING KNEE RAISE	26	51	10 REPETITIONS PER LEG	
PUSH BACK TO THE WALL	39	77	10 REPETITIONS	
DYNAMIC EXTENSION TO THE WALL	33	65	10 REPETITIONS	

DAY 28

DATE: _____

NAME OF THE EXERCISE	EXERCISE	PAGE	REPETITIONS/ DURATION	✓
WALK WHILE LYING DOWN AND THEN BRIDGE	24	47	5 REPETITIONS PER LEG	
HIP THRUST TO THE WALL WITH STATIC STOP	13	25	5 REPETITIONS	
TORSION WITH SUPPORT	1	1	10 REPETITIONS PER SIDE	
SCAPULAR RETRACTION & PROTRACTION	34	67	10 REPETITIONS	
KNEE TO CHEST + KICK BACK	18	35	10 REPETITIONS PER LEG	

TRACKING CHART

DAY	Workout Duration	Physical Feelings	Emotional Feelings	Motivation (high/low)	Are you proud of yourself?
DAY 1					
DAY 2					
DAY 3					
DAY 4					
DAY 5					
DAY 6					
DAY 7					
DAY 8					
DAY 9					
DAY 10					
DAY 11					
DAY 12					
DAY 13					
DAY 14					
DAY 15					
DAY 16					
DAY 17					
DAY 18					
DAY 19					
DAY 20					
DAY 21					
DAY 22					
DAY 23					
DAY 24					
DAY 25					
DAY 26					
DAY 27					
DAY 28					

Made in the USA
Middletown, DE
04 January 2025

68788671R00064